Contents

KU-174-235

Introduction

Introduction

It is a little more than 100 years since Kraepelin began to differentiate manic–depressive illness from what we now call schizophrenia. Slightly more than 50 years ago Cade published his remarkably misreasoned but revolutionary report on lithium treatment of manic excitement, which subsequently helped to launch the field of psychopharmacology. Just 34 years ago, Perris carefully outlined the evidence in favor of using a history of mania to differentiate between bipolar and unipolar subforms of mood disorder. It is just within the past 10 years that the magnitude of the problem of nonresponse or prophylaxis failure with lithium therapy for the average with a polyepisodic course patient has been widely recognized and that other alternatives for the treatment of mania by the United States Food and Drug Administration have begun to be approved.

The 1990s were called the Decade of the Brain. During this period, progress on the identification of likely mechanisms of action of lithium and other mood stabilizers accelerated, but there were not any 'breakthrough' genetic findings. Although there have been people with this disorder for at least as long as humans have been able to describe their experiences with written language, it should be clear that the scientific basis for the treatment of bipolar affective disorder is based on very recent developments.

This book is the result of our collaboration over the past four years to develop and implement evidence-based treatment

Bipolar Disorder
A systematic approach to treatment

Gary S Sachs MD

Director, Bipolar Research Program
Massachusetts General Hospital, and
Assistant Professor of Psychiatry
Harvard Medical School
Boston, MA
USA

Michael E Thase MD

Chief, Division of Adult Academic Psychiatry
Professor of Psychiatry
University of Pittsburgh School of Medicine
Western Psychiatric Institute and Clinic
Pittsburgh, PA
USA

MARTIN DUNITZ

The views expressed in this publication are those
of the authors and not necessarily those of
Martin Dunitz Ltd or any other company.

© Martin Dunitz Ltd 2000

First published in the United Kingdom in 2000 by
Martin Dunitz Ltd
The Livery House
7–9 Pratt Street
London NW1 0AE

Reprinted 2001

Reprinted 2002

A CIP catalogue record for this book is available
from the British Library

ISBN 1-85317-964-7

Composition by Creative Associates, Oxford
Printed and bound in Italy

approaches for mania, bipolar depression and the various other presentations of this pleiomorphic disorder. Beyond this book, our efforts have led to the receipt of a research contract from the National Institute of Mental Health to lead a nationwide, multicenter study of the treatment of bipolar disorder. Although there are necessarily similarities between the approaches described in this book and the *Clinicians' Handbook* we developed for the Systematic Treatment Evaluation Program for Bipolar Disorder (STEP-BD), we wish to make it clear that this book is not a product of that project nor has this book been endorsed by our colleagues at the National Institute of Mental Health.

Our aim is to provide a concise, readily accessible and practical guide to the pharmacotherapy of bipolar disorder, circa 2000. We hope that this will help to reduce the gap (or at times chasm) between what is learned from controlled studies and what is done in everyday clinical practice. To achieve this aim, the scope of coverage was reduced at the expense of a broader review of other treatment modalities. We particularly regret not being able to include descriptions of newer individual-, group- and family-focused psychotherapies for bipolar disorder as these are beginning to gain empirical support (when combined with appropriate pharmacotherapy) after years of relative neglect. We are all too aware that only a fraction of the people with bipolar disorder can be treated effectively with a strict medication model, 'Lithium Clinic'-type approach. We look forward to examining the impact of several intensive psychosocial strategies in the STEP-BD Relapse Prevention and Acute Depression protocols. We have also excluded the more experimental or unconventional medication strategies that ultimately may or may not find their way into the mainstream.

Many people must be acknowledged for their contributions. On the personal level we dedicate this book to our parents (two living, two deceased), wives and children. We wish to thank our mentors and teachers along the way, most particularly David J Kupfer and Jerrold F Rosenbaum.

The labors of our staffs and colleagues on various research projects are most gratefully appreciated. Mike Meakin at Martin Dunitz Ltd must have been 'aged' by at least five years through our perpetual lateness and missed deadlines. Lastly, we thank our patients, who continue to help us to remain in awe of the complexities of brain–behavior relationships and remind us how much more still needs to be learned.

1. An overview of bipolar disorder

The term 'bipolar affective disorder' describes a heterogenous group of conditions characterized by episodes at the two 'poles' of mood disturbance. Mania, a severe state of psychomotor activation and euphoric or irritable mood, defines one pole. Briefer or milder episodes are termed hypomania. The second pole is depression, although perhaps only about 90% of people who have manic episodes will also suffer major depressive episodes. Patients who experience full manic episodes are classified as having the classic or Type 1 form of the illness. Those who experience recurrent depressive episodes and only brief hypomanias are classified as having the Type 2 form of the illness.

The bipolar affective disorder grouping subsumes several other presentations. For example, some episodes are characterized by an admixture of depressive and manic or hypomanic symptoms. These mixed states or mixed bipolar episodes can be both diagnostically challenging and difficult to treat. Another presentation is characterized by a relatively rapid oscillation between depressive and manic or hypomanic episodes. This type of clinical course is called 'rapid cycling'. Although as few as four episodes per year can be called rapid cycling, some patients can experience monthly, weekly or even daily shifts in polarity. As noted above, some individuals experience full manic episodes but apparently never suffer from depression. These so-called, unipolar manias are nevertheless considered to be a Type 1 form of bipolar affective disorder because of similarities in treatment response, family history, phenomenology, and other aspects of clinical course. Conversely, other patients may suffer five or even ten depressive episodes for every one mania. Bipolar episodes often follow a seasonal pattern, with depression more common in the fall (autumn) or winter and mania or hypomania more common in the spring or summer.

Several other mental disorders are closely linked to bipolar affective disorder and probably fall within a broader illness spectrum. 'Cyclothymia' refers to an episodic condition of milder (subsyndromal) or briefer episodes of depression and hypomania. Over time, many, if not most, people with cyclothymia will experience a major depressive episode or full manic episode and hence 'convert' to a bipolar disorder diagnosis. A subset of people with recurrent ('unipolar') depressive episodes also will experience hypomanic or manic episodes over time. On one hand, this reflects the simple fact that the index episode of bipolar disorder may be depression, not mania, and the proper diagnosis is not possible until a manic episode is manifest. On the other hand, Post and others have argued that recurrent depressive episodes may later transduce brain function to increase the probability of experiencing a manic episode. Antidepressants may similarly provoke an initial manic or hypomanic episode in people with recurrent depression. Finally, the diagnosis of schizoaffective disorder includes patients who suffer manic and depressive episodes. These patients do not meet the formal criteria for bipolar affective disorder because of the phenomenology of index episodes (i.e. psychotic features that are too bizarre, disorganized, or mood-incongruent to be grouped confidently within the bipolar family) or persistent psychotic features between affective episodes.

Diagnostic criteria

Table I summarizes the DSM-IV criteria for a manic episode. Note that a hallmark of this approach is the paired requirements that the episode cannot be better accounted for by another psy-

Table I *DSM-IV criteria for a manic episode.*

A.	A distinct period of abnormal and persistent elation or expansive or irritable mood, persisting at least 1 week or requiring hospitalization
B.	During the above, at least three of the following symptoms (four if the mood is only irritable) have been present to a significant degree
1.	Inflated self-esteem or grandiosity
2.	Decreased need for sleep
3.	More talkative than usual or pressure to keep talking
4.	Flight of ideas or racing thoughts
5.	Distractibility
6.	Increase in goal-directed activity or psychomotor agitation
7.	Excessive involvement in pleasurable activities despite potentially painful consequences
D.	Severe impairment, hospitalization or psychosis
E.	The symptoms are not due to substance abuse, a medication effect or a general medical condition

Adapted from the *Diagnostic and Statistical Manual of Mental Disorders*, 4th edn. Copyright © 1994, American Psychiatric Association.

chiatric disorder (e.g. schizophrenia) nor is it likely that the episode is a direct consequence of a general medical disorder or the effect of a mediation or illicit drug intoxication.

Although mania is not, by definition, a psychotic disorder, up to two-thirds of acutely manic individuals will report delusions or hallucinations. Generally, the psychotic features associated with mania are mood congruent, that is, the content of the delusion or impact of the hallucination are consistent with a grandiose or irritable mood. Delusions of grandeur are the most typical examples of mood congruence. Delusions of influence and persecution are not uncommon, however, and the cumulative effects of sleep deprivation, drug and alcohol intoxication, and conflicts with loved ones, employers, mental health providers, or law-enforcement officers may shape or elicit mood incongruent psychotic features.

If not psychotic, the manic individual is prone to overvalued ideas; specifically beliefs, impulsivity, and poor judgement drive indiscretions involving money and relationships, with an apparent lack of appreciation of potentially ruinous consequences.

Not surprisingly, the manic individual often undervalues the need for treatment, and not infrequently, contact with mental health professionals is forced by family or the police. Although this is particularly true for the initial manic episode, even patients with well-established diagnoses and a history of prior treated mania can deny the need for treatment or the validity of the diagnosis in the midst of a manic episode.

Acute mania thus often presents as an emergency and warrants vigorous intervention to both protect the patient and contain the episode. Severe mania can be life-threatening and includes catatonic and delirious presentations that can be diagnostically confusing and result in an overemphasis of antipsychotic medication. If seclusion is necessary, it is important to ensure hydration, stability of vital signs and proper electrolyte balance.

Hypomania is, in essence, an attenuated form of mania. By definition, hypomania is non-psychotic and associated with fewer symptoms and less impairment than a manic episode. Hypomania may progress in severity to mania but, more commonly, it persists for days or weeks at subsyndromal intensity. Of note, hypomania seldom necessitates emergency interventions or the intrusion of others to demand psychiatric care. Rather, the individual may perceive the hypomania as his or her 'best'—a time of optimism, increased speed of thought, decreased need for sleep and heightened productivity. Changes in judgment or risk-taking behavior may result in poor decisions or indiscretions, however, such that this otherwise desirable state is not without adverse consequence.

Table 2 summarizes the criteria of a major depressive episode. These criteria are identical to those used to diagnose the non-bipolar or unipolar forms of depressive disorder. The subtypes or course-modifiers that apply to a major depressive disorder also may be utilized (Table 3). Importantly, major depressive episodes with psychotic features are commonly associated with bipolar disorder, especially among teenagers and younger adults. We consider psychotic depressions prior to age 40 years to convey increased risk for subsequent bipolarity. As noted earlier, a seasonal pattern of recurrent fall (autumn) and winter depressions is common in bipolar disorder, perhaps more so than

Table 2 *DSM-IV criteria for a major depressive episode.*

A. Five (or more) of the following symptoms that persist for at least 2 weeks and result in decreased functioning; including either (1) depressed mood or (2) loss of interest or pleasure

1. Depressed mood most of the day, nearly every day (In children and adolescents, irritable mood can be substituted)

2. Anhedonia (markedly diminished interest or pleasure in all, or almost all, activities)

3. Significant weight loss or weight gain (e.g. an increase or decrease of more than 5% of body weight in a month), or decrease or increase in appetite nearly every day

4. Insomnia or hypersomnia

5. Psychomotor agitation or retardation (observable by others)

6. Fatigue or loss of energy

7. Feelings of worthlessness or inappropriate guilt (can be delusional)

8. Diminished ability to think or concentrate; indecisiveness

9. Recurrent thoughts of suicide or death, including a suicide attempt

B. The symptoms do not meet criteria for a mixed episode (see DSM-IV, p. 335)

C. The symptoms cause significant impairment

D. The symptoms are not due to substance abuse, a medication or a general medical condition

E. The symptoms are not better explained as bereavement (i.e. after the loss of a loved one)

Adapted from the *Diagnostic and Statistical Manual of Mental Disorders*, 4th edn. Copyright © 1994, American Psychiatric Association.

Table 3 *DSM-IV major depressive episode specifiers for bipolar disorder.*

Digit 5 of diagnostic code (296.5X)
1. Mild
2. Moderate
3. Severe (non-psychotic)
4. Severe and psychotic
5. In partial remission
6. In full remission
Narrative (uncoded) specifiers
Atypical features
Catatonic features
Chronic (> 2 years' duration)
Melancholic features
Postpartum onset
Rapid cycling
Seasonal pattern
With/without full interepisode recover

among the non-bipolar depressions. Lastly, although the atypical depression course-modifier is evolved from a different diagnostic tradition independent of the manic depression construct, a relatively large proportion of non-psychotic bipolar depressions are characterized by reverse neurovegetative symptoms, such as oversleeping and weight gain or increased appetite.

Suicidal ideation is common to both bipolar and non-bipolar depressions. Nevertheless, there is some evidence that people with bipolar disorder have a greater risk of violent or potentially lethal suicidal acts, and hence a greater risk of completed suicide. Possible reasons for this increased risk will be discussed later.

Epidemiology

Population surveys consistently document that the lifetime incidence of the Type 1 form of bipolar affective disorder is between 0.8% and 1.2%. Population surveys do not provide an adequate estimate of the prevalence of the Type 2 form of disorder because the methods of case ascertainment are relatively insensitive to detecting milder episodes of hypomania. Working backwards however, it can be estimated that 1–2% of the population have a bipolar Type 2 disorder because 10–20% of patients with 'unipolar' depression have hypomanias.

When compared with schizophrenia, a similarly common but more chronic condition, patients with bipolar affective disorder are more broadly distributed socioeconomically. There is evidence, however, of downward economic drift, particularly among those with more severe, polyepisodic and early-onset forms of bipolar disorder. The incidence of bipolar disorder also appears to be relatively uniform across Western cultures, although the ubiquity of disorder among closed aboriginal cultures has not yet been confirmed.

The Type 1 form of bipolar disorder has a relatively even prevalence among men and women. Thus, when compared with non-bipolar depressive disorders, there is a relative predominance of men. It is possible that this difference in gender distribution reflects a relatively greater contribution of hereditary risk factors in bipolar disorder, with a relative preponderance of psychosocial risk factors (that are more likely to adversely affect women) in non-bipolar depressions. Although probably true, these associations should not be used to reinforce dichotomous thinking: psychosocial stressors are relevant to the course of bipolar disorder and heredity is relevant to dysthymia and major depressive disorder.

Age of first illness onset is another epidemiologic variable that has been used to distinguish between bipolar and non-bipolar forms of mood disorder. Specifically, the initial episode of illness occurs approximately 8–10 years earlier in life in bipolar disorder. An earlier age of onset is generally associated with a greater 'loading' of heritable risk. Evidence emerging over the past decade suggests that the age of onset of both bipolar and non-bipolar mood disorders has decreased. Undoubtedly this is partly an artifact of differences in recognition and treatment-seeking across cohorts. Nevertheless, an initial episode of mania now occurs at an average age of 19 years, and prepubertal illness onset is no longer uncommon.

As in other areas of medicine, an early onset of illness is associated with greater case complexity, episode severity and comorbidity. Adolescent-onset manias are commonly complicated by substance abuse and antecedent histories of conduct or behavioral problems, attention deficit/hyperactivity disorder, and anxiety disorders.

A small but clinically important group will develop mania in late life. This presentation may evolve from a lifetime course of recurrent depression (there is about a 5% risk of mania after three or more episodes of major depression) or it may develop *de novo*. Such patients are more likely to have unrecognized neurological disease or some other systemic general medical illness. Unfortunately, the underlying medication condition may go unrecognized and response to treatment and overall prognosis tends to be poorer in later-onset cases.

Natural history and clinical course

The natural history of bipolar disorder is one of episodes of acute illness followed by periods of complete or nearly complete remission. Generally, a manic episode has a more precipitous onset and a shorter duration than a depressive episode. Mania, for example, has an average episode duration of 4–6 months without treatment. Episodes of bipolar depression generally last

6–9 months. Both types of episode can become chronic (i.e. lasting 2 years or longer), although chronicity is more common for depressive episodes.

Treatment has greatly altered the natural history and, in all likelihood, the phenomenology of bipolar affective disorder. For example, a manic episode generally results in treatment within 1 month, with an average time to response following the onset of treatment of 2–4 weeks. Prompt recognition and treatment of a manic episode, therefore, may reduce ill time by 50%, 75% or even longer. Unfortunately, such an initial response is usually fragile and relapse is common if the intensity of treatment is diminished. This problem is heightened in an era in which acute hospital stays are counted in days rather than weeks or months. Of course, non-adherence is the most likely reason that treatment intensity is reduced. Therefore, it is common in the modern era to document cases in which apparent rapid cycling actually represents a sequence of responses and relapses attributable to a fluctuating level of treatment intensity.

Discontinuation of an effective mood stabilizer also can accelerate the risk of recurrence even after months of stable recovery. Thus, one untoward consequence of effective treatment is the unappreciated risk of increasing the frequency of episodes if the treatment is not complied with or terminated abruptly. A slower reduction of treatment intensity may lessen the risk.

Treatment of bipolar depressive episodes with antidepressants may similarly reduce the length of an average episode by weeks or even months; however, the reduction of the length of the depressive episode may hasten the onset of a hypomanic or manic episode. As illustrated in Figure 1, an 'on again–off again' pattern of antidepressant therapy has been implicated in the genesis of rapid cycling bipolar disorder. Currently, the prevalence of rapid cycling is estimated to be 15–25% in treated populations with bipolar disorder.

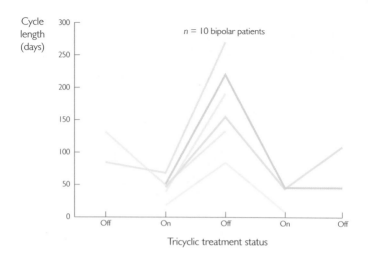

Cycle length (days)

n = 10 bipolar patients

Off   On   Off   On   Off

Tricyclic treatment status

Figure 1 *Tricyclic-induced shortening of the bipolar cycle length (n = 10). Reproduced with permission from Goodwin and Jamison, 1990.*

Although rapid cycling was not unheard of prior to the introduction of antidepressant medications, there is strong evidence that the frequency of this pattern has increased dramatically since the 1960s. Arbitrarily defined by four or more episodes within one calendar year, there are numerous more frequent presentations, including monthly, weekly, and even shorter cycles. Rapid cycling is more common in women (as compared with men) and among those with the bipolar Type 2 pattern. Hypothyroidism is an additional risk factor. Among those with more labile or ultra-rapid cycles there is more diagnostic controversy and borderline personality disorder and related Axis II conditions are important differential considerations.

Across a lifetime, a person with bipolar disorder will suffer an average of eight to ten episodes. About 4–6 years typically separates the first and second episodes, with the interepisode interval typically growing shorter between the second and fifth episodes (Figure 2). Thereafter, the interepisode interval aver-

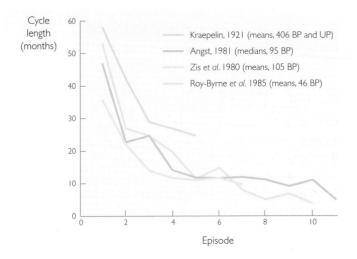

Figure 2 *Average length of episodes across repeated episodes in Type 1 bipolar disorder. Reproduced with permission from Goodwin and Jamison, 1990.*

ages about 18 months. Such averages obscure meaningful individual differences, however, and 10–15 illness-free years are about as common as annual episodes from the outset.

Alcoholism and other forms of substance abuse are both risk factors and consequences of bipolar disorder. Up to 60% of patients will have an alcohol or substance abuse problem at some point. Such comorbidity alters illness course by lengthening episodes and reducing the probability of response to standard theories. Patients with comorbid substance abuse disorders warrant simultaneous treatment with standard psychiatric therapies and chemical dependence counseling and related self-help strategies, i.e. Alcoholics Anonymous (AA) or Narcotics Anonymous (NA).

Bipolar disorder is associated with premature death and reduced life-expectancy. Foremost among risk factors is suicide, which may have a lifetime risk as high as 15–20%. When compared with non-bipolar depression, the higher risk of completed suicide may be attributable to the relatively greater proportion of men (who are more likely to choose lethal means than women), a greater frequency of substance abuse, of psychotic symptoms, or some as yet unidentified neurobiological factor, such as a greater likelihood of serotoninergic dysfunction.

There is less compelling evidence of other health complications that may affect longevity. Factors potentially implicated include increased risk of hypertension, cardiovascular disease and obesity, as well as a high rate of tobacco use. Treatment with lithium, neuroleptics and anticonvulsants increase the risk of weight gain over time and may adversely affect glucose and insulin metabolism. Lithium also may adversely affect renal function over time, although frank cases of kidney failure are fortunately rare.

Family history
Bipolar disorder is associated with increased familial risks of both mania and non-bipolar depression. When compared with the general population, the risk of an affective relative is elevated about four- to five-fold. This increase is at least twice that experienced by the relatives of patients with non-bipolar depression. A similar increase in inherited risk also has been demonstrated by the small number of studies using the 'adopted away' method.

The genetic mechanisms of this increased risk have not yet been elucidated, although a number of loci have been implicated. Polygenetic inheritance is fully consistent with the heterogeneity of the illness.

Studies using twin methods confirm that the inherited risk of monozygotic twins is about three- to four-fold greater than among dizygotic twins. Among monozygous twins, lifetime rates of concordance are above 75%. The risk faced by a dizygous twin is generally not significantly greater than observed among siblings and other first-degree relatives.

Personality and temperament.

There is no single personality or temperament that describes people with bipolar disorder. Prospective studies indicate that episodes of mania and depression inflate ratings of traits such as extroversion or stimulus-seeking and dependence or harm avoidance, respectively. As a result, perceptions of narcissism or melancholic personality types may be shaped by *forms frustes* or early-onset forms of the illness. In any event, an apparent Axis II disorder may certainly complicate the course of bipolar disorder and heighten the need for concomitant psychosocial therapy.

Life events and stress

Although less clearly linked to psychosocial adversity than non-bipolar depression, bipolar disorder is nevertheless affected by life events and social support. For example, a home environment characterized as critical or emotionally charged is associated with a greater risk of relapse. Stressful life events may similarly hasten relapse, either directly by triggering central nervous system stress response system or indirectly via sleep loss or perturbation of the social matrix that helps to entrain biological rhythms.

Suggested reading

Akiskal HS. The prevalent clinical spectrum of bipolar disorders: beyond DSM-IV. *J Clin Psychopharmacol* 1996; **16**: 4S–14S.

American Psychiatric Association. *Diagnostic and Statistical Manual of Mental Disorders*, 4th edn, (DSM-IV). American Psychiatric Association: Washington, DC, 1994.

Angst J. Clinical indications for a prophylactic treatment of depression. *Adv Biol Psychiatry* 1981; **7**: 218–29.

Baldessarini RJ, Tondo L, Faedda GL. Effects of the rate of discontinuing lithium maintenance treatment in bipolar disorders. *J Clin Psychiatry* 1996; **57**: 441–8.

Bauer MS, Dunner DL. Validity of seasonal pattern as a modifier for recurrent mood disorders for DSM-IV. *Comp Psychiatry* 1993; **34**: 159–70.

Goodwin FK, Jamison KR. *Manic–Depressive Illness*. Oxford University Press: New York, 1990.

Howland RH, Thase ME. Cyclothymic disorders. In: Widiger TA, Frances AJ, Pincus HA *et al.*, eds, *DSM-IV Sourcebook*. American Psychiatric Association: Washington, DC, 1995.

Kraepelin E. *Manic–Depressive Insanity and Paranoia*. E&S Livingstone: Edinburgh, 1921.

Perris C. A study of bipolar (manic–depressive) and unipolar recurrent depressive psychoses. *Acta Psychiatr Scand* 1966; **42** (Suppl. 194): 1–188.

Post RM. Transduction of psychosocial stress into the neurobiology of recurrent affective disorder. *Am J Psychiatry* 1992; **8**: 999–1010.

Roy-Byrne P, Post RM, Uhde TW *et al.* The longitudinal course of recurrent affective illness: life chart from research patients at the NIMH. *Acta Psychiatr Scand Suppl* 1985; **317**: 1–34.

Zis AP, Grof P, Webster M, Goodwin FK. Prediction of relapse in recurrent affective disorder. *Psychopharmacol Bull* 1980; **16**: 47–9.

2. Practical treatment of bipolar disorder: a clinician's guide

General approach to treatment

Multiphase treatment strategy

The variability of presentation, course of illness and response to specific treatments requires an iterative approach to treatment. Until more specific treatments become available, reducing the number of trials and errors necessary to find beneficial treatments for individual patients relies on a rational systematic approach to treatment and assessment. The approach to treatment offered in this section is not the only, or necessarily the best, approach but represents one such systematic approach. This general approach for a multiphase treatment strategy is summarized in Figure 3.

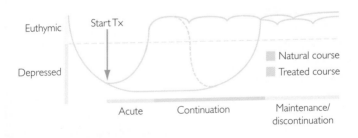

Figure 3 *Multiphase approach to treatment.*

Accurate assessment of mood disorder diagnosis and current episode provides the basis for selecting and staging treatment modalities. Bipolar illness is relatively easy to diagnose when the patient presents with a current manic or mixed episode. Failure to diagnose bipolar illness in a depressed patient is a common occurrence and frequently associated with antidepressant-induced mania. The potential for this poor outcome can be reduced by including in the evaluation of all mood disorder patients, systematic screening for episodes of abnormal mood elevation. By identifying and characterizing the most extreme period of mood elevation, it is possible to determine rapidly whether a patient meets criteria for a diagnosis of a bipolar Type I, bipolar Type II, cyclothymia or a bipolar 'not otherwise specified' (NOS) disorder.

Since the psychiatrist's direct observation of the patient is usually limited to brief interviews, assessment of bipolar patients can be improved by augmenting the patient's clinical report with reports from significant others. Whenever possible, clinicians should endeavor to establish and maintain a positive therapeutic alliance with the patient, their family and any systems important in caring for the patient. With the consent of the patient, establishing a policy of open communication gives the psychiatrist access to the important observations of those who know the patient well. Since a central feature of bipolar illness is episodic distortion in self-assessment, this offers the patient some protection against the risk of relying on their self-observation to guide treatment decisions. As the recipient of multiple inputs, the psychiatrist weighs the conflicting descriptions of the patient's symptoms. The sensitivity and specificity of clinical examination is influenced greatly by the illness and the perspective of the reporter. In general, patient self-report is most sensitive and least specific for symptoms of depression. In contrast, friends and family tend to be most sensitive and least specific for symptoms of mood elevation.

Knowledge of an individual patient's pattern of illness is perhaps the most useful guide to planning treatment, and is especially helpful if episodes are similar in pattern and duration. The use of a graphical mood chart greatly enhances the psychiatrist's ability to recognize patterns of illness and the impact of each treatment. With modest encouragement from the clinician, patients can quickly learn to chart their mood, sleep pattern and treatments on a daily basis (see Appendix A). At follow-up the mood chart can be reviewed and the information incorporated into the patient's chart. Over time, the accumulated mood chart data facilitates tracking of response to treatment, typical precipitants, cycle frequency, pattern of illness and duration of episodes.

Neuropsychiatric assessment

A complete evaluation includes the psychiatric and medical history, physical examination and laboratory investigations. Routine baseline evaluation should include complete blood count, serum chemistries and thyroid functions. Electroencephalogram (EEG), imaging studies and erythrocyte sedimentation rate (ESR) are also reasonable tests to be performed at least once.

Elimination of cycle-promoting agents

Medications that promote cycling, such as antidepressants and any steroid medications, should be eliminated from the treatment regimen whenever possible. Eliminating antidepressants from the treatment regimen appears to be the single most successful intervention for ending rapid cycling. Neuroleptics, particularly phenothiazines, have also been associated with rapid cycling and some patients improve when these agents are discontinued. Our experience suggests that discontinuation of antidepressants often has salutary effects on the cycle rate of non-rapid cycling bipolar illness. Reduction of stimulants (including caffeine) and bronchodilators (albuteral, theophylline, etc.) also appears beneficial.

Encouragement of good mood hygiene

Treatment outcome can be improved in many cases by educating the patient and his or her family about the nature of the illness, encouragement of self-monitoring such as keeping a simple daily mood chart, identifying potential triggers and other principles of good mood hygiene. Although some studies associating environmental events with onset of episodes find little correlation beyond the earliest episodes, most patients are able to learn simple strategies to lessen conflict or avoid precipitants. Advising patients about the need to maintain stable sleep–wake, diet, and exercise schedules, the need to avoid extremes in work, and the need to take care when traveling across time zones is often beneficial. Although, like many of the somatic therapies described later, there are no empirical data showing their effectiveness in treatment refractory bipolar patients, the low cost and low risk associated with these strategies justifies their recommendation.

Since bipolar illness tends to be understood in biological terms, it is interesting that psychotherapy appears beneficial for bipolar patients. No verbal therapies claim acute antimanic benefits but most forms of psychotherapy seem to augment the prophylactic benefit of lithium. While the active elements of psychotherapy remain unclear, the prophylactic efficacy of verbal therapies, as with lithium treatment, appear to require continued treatment.

Among patients receiving lithium prophylaxis for at least 3 years, Priebe et al found a significant association between relapse rates and negative expressed emotion by family members. The impact of negative expressed emotion seems particularly strong in the early phase of an episode and during the period immediately following discharge from the hospital. Mood hygiene can be improved by helping family members to deal constructively with the hostility aroused in relating to the bipolar patient. The impact of expressed emotion may play a role in psychotherapy as well. Numerous anecdotes suggest that during episodes of mania or severe depression insight-oriented therapies can have de-stabilizing effects on mood state. Therapists treating bipolar patients can improve mood hygiene by assessing mood state and making appropriate adjustments to the content, frequency and duration of therapy sessions. As patients become acutely ill, it is most appropriate for sessions to become more frequent but briefer, focusing on safety issues and the control of acute symptoms. Many patients report beneficial experiences from self-help groups such as the National Depressive and Manic Depressive Association (NDMDA).

Diagnosis and treatment of acute episodes

Over the course of bipolar illness, patients may present with acute symptoms diagnosable under DSM-IV criteria as episodes of major depression, mania, hypomania, or mixed episodes. Accurate diagnostic assessment of the current mood state is crucial to choosing an effective intervention. Appendix B provides a systematic format for routine clinical assessement, the 'clinical monitoring form' (CMF) which links eight operationally defined clinical states (Table 4) with the decision-making points in the treatment guidelines offered in this and following sections.

It is often necessary to use non-mood-stabilizing therapies, antidepressants or neuroleptics, for acute- and continuation-phase treatment of depression and mania. Caution should be taken before ruling out the diagnosis of manic or mixed episode, however, since catastrophic consequences may follow the prescription of antidepressants to patients misdiagnosed as suffering from depression who are actually suffering from a manic or mixed episode.

Optimization of mood-stabilizing therapies

After controlling the symptoms in the acute phase, the next treatment priority is preventing recurrence. Using an iterative approach, mood-stabilizing therapies are presented in a stepwise fashion and the impact of each treatment on cycle length is assessed based on follow-up assessment and mood charting. A period equivalent to three times the patient's cycle length and not less than 6 months is usually required for confident determination of prophylactic benefit. Partially effective or ineffective therapies can be discontinued or augmented by adjunctive mood stabilizing agents.

Table 4 *Definitions for assignment of clinical status.*

If DSM criteria for current episode positive		
Episode	Associated symptoms of mania or depression	Assigned status
Major depression*	≥ 5 moderate	Depression
Mania*	≥ 3 moderate	Mania
Hypomania*	≥ 3 moderate	Hypomania
Major depression and mania	≥ 3 moderate for mania and ≥ 5 moderate for depression	Mixed
If DSM criteria for current episode negative		
'Recovered' from last acute episode	Associated symptoms of mania or depression	Assigned status
No	≥ 3 moderate symptoms	Continued symptomatic
No	≤ 2 moderate symptoms	Recovering
Yes, if 'recovering' ≥ 4 consecutive weeks	≤ 2 moderate symptoms	Recovered
Yes	≥ 3 moderate symptoms	Roughening

Implementation of a specific treatment plan

In most cases, a wide range of potential appropriate treatments can be offered to patients. The best way to simplify the treatment options is the use of a treatment algorithm that provides an orderly systematic approach. A general treatment plan can be adapted to individual patients by first selecting a 'menu of reasonable choices' based on the patient's current diagnosis, symptom profile and past history. These reasonable treatments may then be assembled in the sequence most acceptable to the patient. Treatment trials are carried out until clinical objectives are met, the trial is declared ineffective (owing to lack of response at maximal tolerated dose) or adverse effects force a change in treatment. The treatment guidelines presented later in this section illustrate this procedure.

Treatment of psychosis during acute episodes

The risk of adverse effects of neuroleptic such as acute dystonias and tardive dyskinesia, appears to be greater in affectively ill patients. Therefore, neuroleptic exposure should be minimized to the dose necessary to control safely the acute psychotic symptoms within the available resources for patient management. Lithium may have antipsychotic activity apart from its impact on the specific mood disorder component of the illness and might lessen the need for neuroleptic medication. Use of anticonvulsants and benzodiazepines also appears to lessen the need for neuroleptic medication. Nonetheless, bipolar patients with psychotic depression or psychotic mania typically require treatment with neuroleptic medication, although patients with milder symptoms may be treated appropriately with mood-stabilizing agents alone or in combination with antidepressants. Following resolution of the acute psychotic symptoms and an appropriate continuation phase, neuroleptic medications can be tapered gradually.

In the absence of data specific to treatment of affective psychosis, the approach to treatment may be guided by experience with unipolar delusional depression, where the combination of an antidepressant and antipsychotic medications may be more effective than either agent alone. In most cases, treatment of psychotic mania would consist of mood-stabilizing medication in combination with a neuroleptic whereas treatment of most bipolar depressions with psychotic features would comprise a mood stabilizer, a neuroleptic and an antidepressant medication. The presence of psychotic features appears to increase the likelihood of treatment resistance. In cases where the immediate need to control psychotic symptoms takes clear precedence over specific treatment for depression or mania, initiation of antipsychotic therapy or electroconvulsive therapy (ECT) precedes other interventions.

Indications for non-standard treatments

In any of the variety of circumstance in which use of non-standard or innovative treatments (Table 5) may be appropriate, care should be taken to document the indication in medical records and to ensure that the patient is aware when non-standard treatment is administered. The indication for non-standard treatment initiated by the clinician is strongest for patients who have severe episodes refractory to multiple standard treatments. Adjunctive use of innovative treatments known to be compatible with standard treatments is also generally preferred prior to use of unproven treatments in place of those with known safety and efficacy.

Specific treatment strategies

The general approach already outlined enables the psychiatrist to choose an appropriate and specific strategy for a patient's cir-

Table 5   *Indications for innovative treatment.*

Indication	Example
Standard treatments have failed	Use of stimulant after non-response to more than one standard antidepressant
Standard treatments are intolerable	Use of DHEA in patient with a history of severe headache during prior treatment with multiple standard agents with different mechanisms/structure
Innovative treatment compatible with standard treatment	Patient requests adjunctive use of omega-3 fatty acids
Standard treatments are unacceptable	Patient refuses standard treatments because of fears based on knowledge of individuals with unfavorable outcome

cumstances. Choice of initial treatment strategy is based on the priority given to the need to treat the current acute episode versus altering the rate of cycling. Simple guidelines are presented in subsequent chapters for acute mania, bipolar depression, mixed episodes and rapid cycling. There are several dimensions involved in the progression of steps outlined in these guidelines. The guidelines present a sequence of treatment categories and each category lists a sequence of individual agents. Phase of treatment is another important dimension of treatment strategy over time because treatment adjustments are needed to meet the different goals and problems of each phase.

The treatment phases defined by Kupfer and Frank for unipolar illness can also be applied to bipolar illness. Separate consideration of patient needs during the acute, continuation and maintenance phases adds clarity to the complex task of treatment planning (Figure 4). Each algorithm places acute-phase therapies on the horizontal dimension and prophylactic strategies on the vertical axis.

Acute-phase treatment

The acute phase begins when the patient meets criteria for an episode (depression, mania, hypomania or mixed) and treatment is initiated. Each individual acute treatment trial is carried out to one of three endpoints:

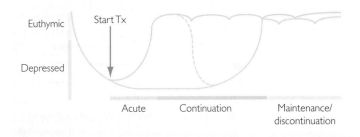

Figure 4 *Disease course: comparison of multiphase treatment compared with no treatment.*

1. Discontinuation because the patient is unable to tolerate adverse effects of treatment.
2. Discontinuation because the patient has failed to respond to a maximal trial of the treatment (including, if warranted, augmentation strategies).
3. The patient has improved during this treatment.

Problems during the acute phase include treatment intolerance, inadequate dosage, partial response and non-response. Treatments are adjusted or replaced as necessary to manage these problems until the acute symptoms remit ending the acute phase.

Continuation-phase treatment

Remission of acute symptoms defines the beginning of the continuation phase, but relapse with full or partial return of symptoms is the most frequently encountered problem during the continuation phase. Successful acute therapies are therefore continued at full dosage for a period of time to prevent relapse. With the remission of symptoms, the continuation phase is also a time when denial of illness fosters non-adherence.

The length of the continuation phase is based on the clinician's estimate of the period necessary to exceed the likely (natural) duration of episode in the absence of treatment. Whether the estimated duration of the continuation phase is determined on the basis of the patient's prior episodes or based on a more general estimate of the likely duration of depressive or manic episodes, the purpose of the continuation phase is to avoid relapse. This is most often accomplished by maintaining treatment at the levels required to induce remission but may involve titration of the dosage. Some treatment-responsive patients may benefit by dose reduction during the continuation phase if medication side-effects substantially negate the gains from remission of mood symptoms. A larger group will intermittently experience significant symptoms (continued symptomatic) during the continuation phase, and while not fulfilling criteria for an acute depressive episode, these may warrant an increase in antidepressant (or antimanic) treatments.

The continuation phase ends and the discontinuation phase or maintenance phase begins when the patient has been in remission for eight consecutive weeks and is declared to have recovered from the acute episode.

Discontinuation-phase/Maintenance-phase treatment

The discontinuation phase follows a decision to discontinue a treatment and involves monitoring for recurrence while gradually tapering medication.

A decision to redirect the therapeutic focus away from treatment of the acute episode toward maintaining recovery or preventing the recurrence of future acute episodes launches the maintenance phase. Many patients experience intermittent subsyndromal symptoms (roughening) during the discontinuation or maintenance phase. The significance of roughening depends on whether it is the harbinger of an impending acute episode or is merely a brief period of mild symptoms with little clear relation to the patient's mood disorder. Studies of such interepisode symptoms performed by Keller and by Fava suggest that roughening with features of depression often resolves without intervention. Symptoms of hypomania carry a higher risk of evolving into full affective episodes.

After the patient has recovered, the occurrence of symptoms meeting criteria for an acute episode would be considered a recurrence (new episode) requiring reintroduction of acute treatments.

How long should maintenance therapy continue? There is considerable debate as to when lifetime prophylaxis should be recommended. This complex debate need not impede most routine treatment since, in many important areas, there is broad consensus among experts. Expert consensus supports at least 1 year of prophylaxis following the first manic episode and any subsequent manic episode. There is also general agreement that patients with three or more episodes warrant long-term maintenance therapy.

Selection of specific agents

At present no symptom or laboratory profiles have been found that allow selection of medication on the basis of predictable markers of response. In the absence of these predictors, drugs can be selected on the basis of known personal or family history of response, the need to treat comorbid conditions, matching adverse effect profiles to ameliorate acute target symptoms, or strong patient preference.

Even in cases where other selection factors are likely determinants of treatment selection (e.g. the patient's mother responded to doxepin), it is useful to discuss risks and side-effect profiles in the context of the other choices the treating psychiatrist might deem reasonable for an individual patient. Better informed patients who know what to expect from medications they have been involved in choosing are likely to find it easier to maintain fidelity to their treatment plan.

The practical tables in this book are intended to be used as an aide when discussing with patients which medications the clinician regards as the most reasonable choices for an individual. Generally it is useful to review the information in the practical table, encourage the patient to participate in selecting from the reasonable choices and provide a copy of the relevant table for the patient.

Initiation of treatment

Once selected, priority should be given to initiating treatment in a manner that anticipates problems that might lead the patient to disqualify a treatment selected as the most desirable. Patient and family education is the best means of avoiding this early stumbling block. The authors recommend reviewing the data with the patient, together with the available support with emphasis on the intended initial dosage, time of administration, expectable side-effects, and which adverse experiences should trigger additional contact with the clinician.

Where multiple forms of the same medication are available, it is more desirable to begin treatment with the form likely to be best tolerated rather than switching to the better-tolerated form after adverse effects occur. Split dosing can also be employed as required to enhance tolerability but adherence drops with multiple daily dosing and once-daily dosing is most desirable. Similarly, initial doses may need to be lowered from those recommended for elderly patients and those with greater sensitivity to particular adverse effects.

In conclusion, a flow-chart showing treatment of acute episodes and relapse prevention pathways is shown in Figure 5.

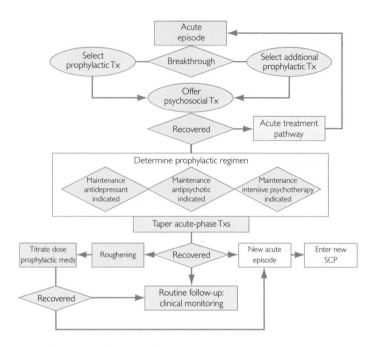

Figure 5 *Integrated acute and relapse-prevention pathways.*

Suggested reading

American Psychiatric Association. Practice guideline for the treatment of patients with bipolar disorder. *Am J Psychiatry* 1994; **151**: 1–36.

Basco MR, Rush AJ. *Cognitive–Behavioral Therapy for Bipolar Disorder*. The Guilford Press: New York, 1996.

Bauer MS, McBride L, Chase C *et al*. Manual-based group psychotherapy for bipolar disorder: a feasibility study. *J Clin Psychiatry* 1998; **59**: 449–55.

Frank E, Prien RF, Jarrett RB *et al*. Conceptualization and rationale for consensus definitions of terms in major depressive disorder. Remission, recovery, relapse, and recurrence. *Arch Gen Psychiatry* 1991; **48**: 851–5.

Frank E, Kupfer DJ, Ehlers CL et al. Interpersonal and social rhythm therapy for bipolar disorder: Integrating interpersonal and behavioral approaches. Behav Therapist 1994; 17: 143–9.

Frank E, Hlastala S, Ritenour A et al. Inducing lifestyle regularity in recovering bipolar disorder patients: results from the maintenance therapies in bipolar disorder protocol. Biol Psychiatry 1997; 41: 1165–73.

Frank E, Swartz HA, Mallinger AG et al. Adjunctive psychotherapy for bipolar disorder: effects of changing treatment modality. J Abnorm Psychol 1999; 108: 579–87.

Goodwin FK, Jamison KR. Manic–Depressive Illness. Oxford University Press: New York, 1990.

Kanas N. Group psychotherapy with bipolar patients: a review and synthesis (review). Int J Group Psychother 1993; 43: 321–33.

Keller MB, Lavori PW, Kane JM et al. Subsyndromal symptoms in bipolar disorder. A comparison of standard and low serum levels of lithium. Arch Gen Psychiatry 1992; 49: 371–6.

Miklowitz DJ. Psychotherapy in combination with drug treatment for bipolar disorder. J Clin Psychopharmacology 1996; 16 (Suppl. 1): 56S–66S.

Miklowitz DJ, Goldstein MJ, Doane JA et al. Is expressed emotion an index of a transactional process? I. Parents' affective style. Fam Process 1989; 28: 153–67.

Miklowitz DJ, Frank E, George EL. New psychosocial treatments for the outpatient management of bipolar disorder. Psychopharmacol Bull 1996; 32: 613–21.

Nilsson A. Lithium therapy and suicide risk. J Clin Psychiatry 1999; 60 (Suppl. 2): 85–8; discussion 111–16.

Priebe S, Wildgrube C, Muller-Oerlinghausen B. Lithium prophylaxis and expressed emotion. Br J Psychiatry 1989; 154: 396–9.

Sachs GS. Bipolar mood disorder: practical strategies for acute and maintenance phase treatment. J Clin Psychopharmacol 1996; 16 (Suppl. 1): 32S–47S.

Sachs GS, Printz DJ, Kahn DA et al. The Expert Consensus Guideline Series: Medication Treatment of Bipolar Disorder 2000. Postgrad Med 2000; April (special no.): 1–104.

Van Gent EM, Vida SL, Zwart FM. Group therapy in addition to lithium therapy in patients with bipolar disorders. Acta Psychiatr Belg 1988; 88: 405–18.

3. Treatment for mood elevation: hypomania, mania and mixed states

The separate criteria provided in the DSM-IV classification for diagnosing hypomania, mania and mixed episodes imply that these are distinct conditions. In clinical practice, however, boundaries between them are unreliable. All three states share common features of abnormally elevated mood and associated features of hypervigilance, reactivity, restlessness, agitation and aggression (Figure 6) and are differentiated based on the extent to which symptoms of depression are present and the degree of functional impairment caused by the episode. Bipolar Type I

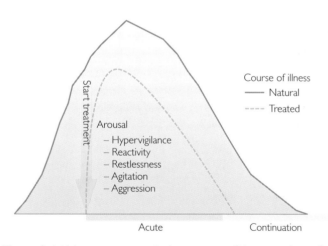

Figure 6 *Initial target symptoms in the treatment of the acute phase of mania.*

patients commonly exhibit a course that fluctuates between these states in a progression that is seemingly orderly at times and at other times chaotic. Therefore, except where otherwise indicated, all statements here concerning treatment for mania should be considered to apply to any episode of mood elevation in a bipolar Type I patient.

The characteristic that most frequently differs between episodes of depression and mood elevation is the variability of the symptoms over time. Even flagrantly manic patients may have hours or days with no overt symptomatology. Since, in many cases, mood elevation is better characterized as a state of hyper-reactivity rather than hyperactivity, assessment in a low-stimulus office setting is likely to be unrevealing. This and the fact that the most common complaint during episodes of mania is 'depression' makes diagnostic confidence in ruling out the presence of current mania on the basis of brief interviews very low. Careful assessment and collateral sources can reduce the risk of misdiagnosis and mistreatment.

Initiation of treatment

Following recognition of a new episode of abnormal mood elevation, six basic clinical decisions should be confronted (Figure 7).

The first steps in treatment of mania are to ensure saftey, to eliminate cycle-promoting agents and to initiate specific antimanic therapies. Along with discontinuing antidepressant medications, consideration should be given to eliminating any other agents that have been implicated as causing mania (e.g. steroids, stimulants, sympathomimetics, hormones, muscle relaxants, triazolobenzodiazepines).

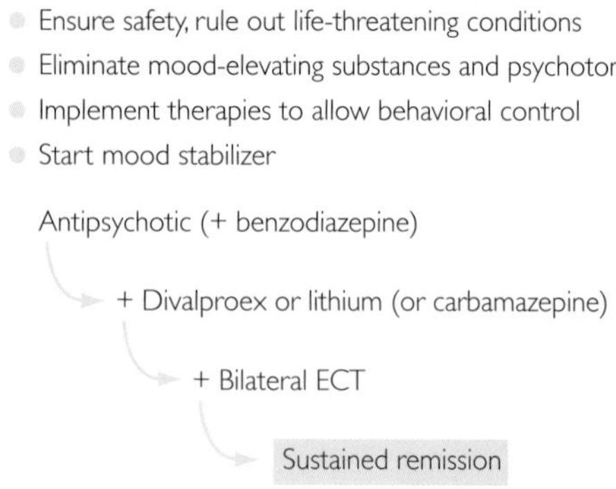

- Ensure safety, rule out life-threatening conditions
- Eliminate mood-elevating substances and psychotomimetics
- Implement therapies to allow behavioral control
- Start mood stabilizer

Antipsychotic (+ benzodiazepine)

   → + Divalproex or lithium (or carbamazepine)

      → + Bilateral ECT

        → | Sustained remission |

Figure 7 *Clinical strategy in the treatment of the acute phase of mania.*

Ensuring safety and restoring behavioral control

In all but the mildest cases, acute manic and mixed episodes warrant hospitalization to ensure the patient's safety at the initiation of treatment. Even in the absence of complications arising from possible general medical conditions, the hyperarousal and impulsivity that typifies acute mania poses a serious threat to the patient and those around them. Simple retreat from an uncontrolled, high-stimulus environment to the buffered interactions of the hospital often reduces overt symptom expression. A state of low symptom expression is a highly desirable context for starting medical treatment, but any lull in acute symptoms is precarious and must not be mistaken for recovery. The presence of staff and family members who are skilled in the art of avoiding confrontation while redirecting behavior, ignoring provocation where possible, delaying potentially problematic interactions (e.g. phone calls from business associates) and distracting from ungratified urges, are particularly valuable assets during the lag between initiation of medical treatment and the onset of anti-manic effects.

Given the premium on rapid symptom reduction, most acutely ill inpatients will benefit from beginning treatment with an antipsychotic agent in combination with divalproex, lithium or carbamazepine. Atypical antipsychotic agents and divalproex have the advantage of being generally well-tolerated even at high doses used to achieve therapeutic levels within the first 24 hours. Benzodiazepines may also offer a relatively safe adjunct to the anti-arousal regime but high doses can lead to counterproductive disinhibition.

Discharge from the hospital is appropriate once sufficient behavioral control is achieved to allow safe management, given the available resources for outpatient treatment. With reasonably aggressive treatment, this degree of symptomatic improvement may be achievable within 1–4 weeks. From the point of initial improvement to sustained full symptomatic recovery from the episode, however, generally requires an additional interval of 12–24 weeks and functional recovery is often delayed for longer than 1 year.

Selection of antimanic mood stabilizer

Preference should be given to agents with established antimanic efficacy therefore, the acute mania pathway (Figure 8) begins with either lithium, divalproex, carbamazepine and/or an antipsychotic medication, haloperidol, olanzapine, or risperidone. Use of these treatments in combination is recommended before moving on to other putative antimanic agents. ECT has also been shown to be effective treatment for mania and is available for refractory cases and when patient preference or symptom acuity dictates use of the most rapidly effective treatment available. A few reports suggesting worsening of acute mania during treatment with unilateral non-dominant ECT provides a rationale for use of bilateral ECT when treating mania.

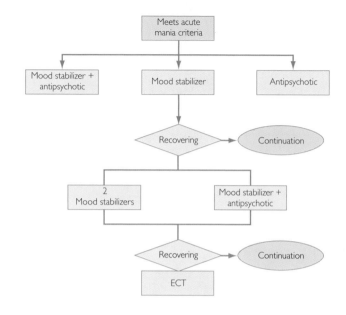

Figure 8 *Acute mania pathway.*

Use of other antimanic agents

Should the first-line agent prove ineffective or unacceptable, the next tier of treatment consists of lamotrigine, topiramate, or clozapine, agents with at least one multicenter controlled study with an adequate sample indicating antimanic efficacy. Requirement for slow titration is less of a limitation when using these agents for refractory mania, where rapidity of response is less of a concern. Despite reports of excellent response in refractory patients, the use of clozapine is limited by concern about bone marrow suppression and the indefinite requirement for blood monitoring.

In addition, adrenergic blocking agents and calcium channel-blocking agents may be considered; results of small studies found the agents clonidine and verapamil to be equivalent to lithium. Uncontrolled case series report the antimanic benefit of cholinomimetics (e.g. choline and donepezil), other anticonvulsants (e.g. gabapentin, acetazolamide and tiagabine), and other antipsychotics. Given the seriousness of acute mania, these and other non-standard treatments are best held in reserve for refractory cases or used as adjuncts to treatments with established efficacy.

Considerations for special subpopulations

Current hypomania

Patients with current hypomania and no prior history of mania or mixed episodes may be managed less aggressively on an outpatient basis. Absence of prior severe episodes does not assure against progression to mania. The need to watch for impending mania is present for mood disorder patients of all types but those with bipolar Type I relatives are likely to be most at risk. Warning the patient and significant others about potential signs of progression to mania can create opportunities to truncate impending episodes and avoid the consequences of uncontrolled mania.

Psychosis

Psychosis (e.g. hallucinations, delusions, or formal thought disorder) and extreme agitation are clear signs for aggressive treatment. Lithium alone has modest benefit in these cases. Antipsychotics are clearly indicated as part of the initial treatment and appear to be more rapidly effective than lithium and possibly other putative mood stabilizers. Anticonvulsants (except carbamazepine and lamotrigine) can often be titrated rapidly.

Current substance abuse

Substance abuse is common among patients presenting with acute mania. While in some instances the manic episode may truly be substance induced, this possiblity need not delay initiation of antimanic treatment. Patients who remain symptomatic for longer than 72 hours after testing negative for illicit substances are likely to have primary mania. Withdrawal syndromes can also complicate the course of recovery.

The elderly
Elderly patients may experience intolerance when treated with standard doses of antimanic medications. Antimanic benefit also tends to be achieved at serum levels lower than those required by younger adults.

Euphoric mania
Pure euphoric mania is unusual and likely to respond best to lithium.

Mania with depressive features
Mania with depressive features short of full depressive episodes appears to be more responsive to divalproex or carbamazepine than to lithium. No treatment is clearly superior to placebo for patients with full mixed episodes, but expert opinion favors the use of an anticonvulsant-type mood stabilizer over lithium. The presence of dysphoria is not an indication for standard antidepressant medication unless the dysphoria persists at least 2 weeks beyond full resolution of hypomanic symptoms.

Course of acute treatment

Whichever initial medical treatment is chosen, the immediate goal of titration to therapeutic range is followed by titration to clinical effect. In practice, this requires a periodic evaluation of the patient's progress to determine whether further increases should be made in dosing or if additional treatment should be added to the regime. The timing of patient assessment remains a matter of clinical judgment. In the absence of response, it may be impractical to delay augmenting the acute treatment regime;

however, assessing the benefit of any treatment based on periods less than 1 week risks creating a false impression of response as well as non-response.

Manic patients typically tolerate reasonably aggressive treatment surprisingly well, although when manic symptoms remit, complaints of adverse effects increase. In some cases, this phenomenum corresponds to an alteration in serum drug levels while in others, it probably reflects a state-dependent variation in perception. In either case, the alteration of dose or contra-active intervention is frequently necessary to avoid early rejection of treatment.

Each treatment introduced in the acute phase should be continued with upward titration and monitoring of response every 3–14 days. If the treatment is intolerable or the patient fails to respond to a maximal dose, patients also remain in the acute mania pathway and the next most attractive treatment on the menu of reasonable choices is added.

Endpoints

As illustrated in Chapter 5, Figure 10, patients may remain in the acute mania pathway until reaching the criteria for recovery. Patients meeting the criteria for depression in the absence of manic symptoms enter the acute depression pathway, while continuing antimanic therapies.

Suggested reading

Bowden CL, Brugger AM, Swann AC et al. Efficacy of divalproex vs lithium and placebo in the treatment of mania. The Depakote Mania Study Group. *JAMA* 1994; **271**: 918–24; published erratum appears in *JAMA* 1994; **271**: 1830.

Bowden CL, Janicak PG, Orsulak P et al. Relation of serum valproate concentration to response in mania. *Am J Psychiatry* 1996; **153**: 765–70.

Freeman MP, Stoll AL. Mood stabilizer combinations: a review of safety and efficacy. *Am J Psychiatry* 1998; **155**: 12–21.

Janicak PG, Levy NA. Rational copharmacy for acute mania. *Psychiatr Ann* 1998; **28**: 204–12.

Keck PE Jr, McElroy SL, Strakowski SM. Anticonvulsants and antipsychotics in the treatment of bipolar disorder. *J Clin Psychiatry* 1998; **59** (Suppl. 6): 74–81.

Suppes T, McElroy SL, Gilbert J et al. Clozapine in the treatment of dysphoric mania. *Biol Psychiatry* 1992; **32**: 270–80.

Swann AC, Bowden CL, Morris D et al. Depression during mania: treatment response to lithium or divalproex. *Arch Gen Psychiatry* 1997; **54**: 37–42.

Tohen M, Sanger TM, McElroy SL et al. Olanzapine versus placebo in the treatment of acute mania. Olanzapine HGEH Study Group. *Am J Psychiatry* 1999; **156**: 702–9.

4. Treatment of bipolar depression

Treatment of bipolar depression represents a common clinical dilemma for clinicians. Compared with unipolar depression, bipolar depression is associated with a lower treatment response rate and a higher suicide rate. While these factors are compelling reasons to administer aggressive treatment, 31–70% of depressed bipolar patients treated with standard antidepressants alone will experience treatment-emergent hypomania or mania. To reduce this risk, expert consensus supports miminizing the patient's exposure to standard antidepressants, and when standard antidepressant medications are prescribed the co-administration of lithium or another mood-stabilizing medication is always recommended.

Following recognition of a new episode of bipolar depression, the treating psychiatrist and patient confront the eight basic clinical decision points summarized in Table 6.

Considerations for special subpopulations

The subpopulation of **treatment-naïve** bipolar Type I and bipolar Type II patients includes a substantial proportion of patients with good prognoses who are likely to respond well to mood-stabilizers. Patients with a history of prior treatment suffering a recurrence during an interval in which they received no prophylactic treatment are also frequently responsive to treatment with mood stabilizers.

Table 6 *Clinical decision points following recognition of a new episode of bipolar depression.*

Initial decision points	Suggested starting point
1. Initiate/Optimize Mood Stabilizer	Review mood-stabilizer menu of reasonable choices
2. Determine intensity of psychosocial intervention	Select from available psychotherapeutic resources or routine clinical care*
3. Determine indication for standard antidepressant medication	Review antidepressant menu of reasonable choices
4. Determine indication for ECT	Review indications for ECT
5. Determine indication for antipsychotic medication	Review indication for antipsychotic medication
6. Determine indication for non-standard treatment	Review indications for non-standard treatments and innovative treatment menu
7. Determine appropriate follow-up interval	Schedule follow-up
8. Determine quantity of medication to be dispensed	Review potential for overdose, drug interactions, safety in overdose and alternatives for dispensing medication

Patients with breakthrough episodes occurring during mood-stabilizer maintenance therapy appear to be less treatment-responsive, particularly if the breakthrough occurred while receiving therapeutic levels of lithium, valproate, or carbamazepine. Such patients may, however, respond to an increased dose of their prophylactic treatment of mood-stabilizer therapy, particularly if their mood-stabilizing agent was maintained at suboptimal levels (lithium <0.8 mmol/l, valproate <80 μg/ml, or carbamazepine <8.0 μg/ml).

Breakthrough episodes occurring during the course prophylaxis with mood stabilizer and antidepressant therapy may represent an even more refractory subgroup but might also include some cases in which the course of illness was driven by the antidepressant itself. For these patients, acute treatment recommendations follow the same guideline (increase dose or add a new antidepressant) but following an appropriate period of continuation treatment, antidepressant medication would be tapered (in the maintenance phase).

Patients with a history of treatment-emergent affective switch or rapid cycling are at highest risk of treatment emergent switch or cycle acceleration when treated with standard antidepressants.

Selection of mood stabilizer

Experts generally recommend a mood stabilizer as initial treatment for bipolar depression regardless of subtype because, when this class of medication is effective, the risks associated with antidepressant use can be avoided. Moreover, mood stabilizers appear to be effective for most bipolar depressed patients. Although published reports suggest each of the 'mood stabilizers' is effective at least in open use, the case for lithium is most compelling, with eight controlled trials showing lithium superior to placebo for bipolar depression. In fact, the only methodologically sound trial available that compared a mood stabilizer alone with mood stabilizer and antidepressant found no benefit of the combination over lithium alone. Even when ineffective, treatment with a mood stabilizer can reduce the potential risk of affective switch that is associated with concomitant antidepressant use by approximately 50%.

In the majority of cases, over the first 3 weeks of treatment, it is reasonable to offer patients with bipolar depression mood-stabilizer medications. If the patient is not substantially improved at that point, standard antidepressants or ECT should be offered unless contraindicated based on individual history.

Selection of antidepressant medication

The menu of reasonable choices (Figure 9) offered for standard antidepressant therapy recognizes the overall efficacy of approved standard antidepressant medication to be equivalent and that specific contraindications (e.g. allergy, cardiac status, insurance restrictions, cost, safety in overdose) require eliminating some choices in individual cases. The menu gives the designation first-line antidepressant to those drugs with the most desirable adverse-effect profile (i.e. the likelihood of serious adverse effects very low, and the risk of tolerability of expectable adverse effects very high).

ECT and treatments with mechanisms of action similar to first-line agents but with less desirable adverse-effect profiles are designated as 'available if preferred'.

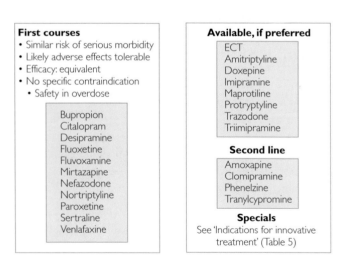

First courses
- Similar risk of serious morbidity
- Likely adverse effects tolerable
- Efficacy: equivalent
- No specific contraindication
  - Safety in overdose

Bupropion
Citalopram
Desipramine
Fluoxetine
Fluvoxamine
Mirtazapine
Nefazodone
Nortriptyline
Paroxetine
Sertraline
Venlafaxine

Available, if preferred

ECT
Amitriptyline
Doxepine
Imipramine
Maprotiline
Protryptyline
Trazodone
Triimipramine

Second line

Amoxapine
Clomipramine
Phenelzine
Tranylcypromine

Specials
See 'Indications for innovative treatment' (Table 5)

Figure 9 *Antidepressant menu of reasonable choices.*

Indications for non-standard treatments

The availability of standard agents with differing structures, adverse-effect profiles and mechanisms provides a long list of therapeutic agents, that can be offered with confidence before using non-standard treatment. There is little to be gained, however, by forbidding patients to use adjuncts such as dietary supplements with no known contraindication.

Indications for ECT

ECT may be appropriate at any time, including as an initial treatment when dictated by symptom acuity or patient preference. All patients should be made aware of its availability. ECT may be encouraged as an early option for acutely suicidal, psychotic, catatonic or severely depressed patients but is generally held in reserve for patients intolerant of, or refractory to, mood stabilizers and standard antidepressant medications.

Indications for antipsychotic medication

Patients with delusions, hallucinations and severe agitation often benefit from adjunctive antipsychotic medications. Atypical antipsychotic medication may improve some symptoms of depression but there is not data as yet suggesting that these agents have antidepressant properties comparable with standard antidepressant medications. Conventional antipsychotic medications, particularly at high doses, can increase dysphoria in some patients.

Follow-up intervals

Local standards and clinician judgment determine acceptable intervals for follow-up. In most circumstance, when new medical treatment is initiated, a follow-up interval of 1–2 weeks is appropriate for managing most outpatients. Patients with mild–moderate depression and good support systems may be managed more safely at longer intervals than severely ill patients who lack reliable supports; however all depressed patients are at risk of self-destructive behavior. In the absence of reliable predictors of the danger, it makes sense to evaluate both inclination and opportunity for self-harm. Patients with active suicidal ideation or other signs of high inclination warrant aggressive treatment aimed at reducing the depression, and may require hospitalization since none of the currently available antidepressant treatments for outpatients delivers reliable results in less than 3 weeks. If measures are taken to monitor adequately the patient and reduce opportunities for self-harm (for example, by eliminating access to firearms and other lethal agents), many acutely depressed patients can be managed without hospitalization. Accordingly, it is best to initiate treatment with a follow-up interval that avoids dispensing large amounts of potentially lethal medications (especially lithium and tricyclic antidepressants).

Quantity of medication to be dispensed

Depression is a risk factor for suicide, even in patients showing no current self-destructive urges. Limiting the quantity of medication prescribed at any one time to amounts that would not be lethal if the entire amount dispensed were ingested does not, by itself, assure safety but can lessen one potential source of lethality. Dispensing amounts of medication sufficient to ensure supply to the next appointment may require extra safety measures.

Acute-phase management

The goal of follow-up visits during the acute phase is to monitor response and manage adverse effects. Figure 7 illustrates decision-making over a typical course of acute treatment. When patients present with remission of depression it is appropriate to offer continuation treatment (see Chapter 1). Similarly, it may be wisest to make no changes in the treatment for patients with substantial improvement (>30%) even though their clinical status remains 'depressed' or 'continues to be symptomatic'.

Reports from Nierenberg and Fava suggest a progressively lower conditional probability of response given no significant improvement after 2, 4, 6, and 8 weeks of treatment at a given dose of antidepressant medication. Therefore, patients experiencing no significant improvement and no significant adverse effects are candidates for upward dose titration until, maximum tolerated doses are achieved. When adverse effects preclude increasing dosage, titration is delayed or dosage may be decreased to allow management of adverse effects. If these precautions do not succeed in allowing an adequate treatment trial, alternative treatment may be required.

Endpoints

As illustrated in Figures 1 and 2, acute-phase treatment continues unless the patient experiences affective switch (hypomania, mania, mixed episode) or recovery. Patients unable to tolerate an effective dosage or who are unresponsive to a full trial of maximal dosage, are offered acute treatment with another standard antidepressant, ECT or innovative treatment, depending on their symptom acuity and history of prior response.

Before concluding that a treatment is ineffective, some experts recommend augmentation strategies such as lithium, thyroid, stimulants, or neurotransmitter precursors in an effort to potentiate standard treatments. The benefit of these agents is not well established but augmentation strategies may be beneficial even if their usefulness is limited to sustaining therapeutic optimism long enough to complete a 16-week therapeutic trial with the highest tolerated dose of a standard agent.

Management of affective switch begins with discussing the risk of switch and warning signs with patients and family members. There is no data to guide management of affective switch but reduction or elimination of antidepressant medication may suffice in mild cases. Treatment is otherwise the same as primary hypomania or mania.

Transition to continuation-phase treatment begins when the patient is assigned a clinical status of recovering; however the transition from recovering to recovered seldom occurs smoothly. For most patients the early months typically include weeks in which the assigned clinical status will be 'continues symptomatic' or 'depressed'. Such 'relapses' are to be expected and, when persistent, may indicate a need for further titration of the acute-phase treatment.

Suggested reading

Altshuler LL, Post RM, Leverich GS et al. Antidepressant-induced mania and cycle acceleration: a controversy revisited. *Am J Psychiatry* 1995; **152**: 1130–8.

Avery D, Winokur G. The efficacy of electroconvulsive therapy and antidepressants in depression. *Biol Psychiatry* 1976; **12**: 507–23.

Calabrese J, Bowden C, Sachs G et al. A double-blind placebo-controlled study of lamotrigine monotherapy in outpatients with bipolar I depression. *J Clin Psychiatry* 1999; **60**: 79–88.

Cohn JB, Collins G, Ashbrook E et al. A comparison of fluoxetine, imipramine and placebo in patients with bipolar depressive disorder. *Int Clin Psychopharmacol* 1989; **4**: 313–14.

Himmelhoch JM, Thase ME, Mallinger AG et al. Tranylcypromine versus imipramine in anergic bipolar depression. *Am J Psychiatry* 1991; **148**: 910–16.

Hlastala SA, Frank E, Mallinger AG et al. Bipolar depression: an underestimated treatment challenge. *Depress Anxiety* 1997; **5**: 73–83.

Kukopulos A, Reginaldi D, Laddomada P et al. Course of the manic–depressive cycle and changes caused by treatment. *Pharmakopsychiatr Neuropsychopharmakol* 1980; **13**: 156–67.

Mendels J. Lithium in the treatment of bipolar depression. *Am J Psychiatry* 1976; **133**: 373–8.

Mendels J, Secunda SK, Dyson WL. A controlled study of the anti-depressant effects of lithium carbonate. *Arch Gen Psychiatry* 1972; **26**: 154–7.

Nemeroff C, Evans D, Gyulai L *et al.* A double-blind, placebo-controlled comparison of imipramine and paroxetine in the treatment of bipolar depression. *Am J Psychiatry* (in press).

Sachs GS, Lafer B, Stoll AL *et al.* A double-blind trial of bupropion versus desiprimine for bipolar depression. *J Clin Psychiatry* 1994; **55**: 391–3.

Wehr TA, Goodwin FK. Can antidepressants cause mania and worsen the course of affective illness? *Am J Psychiatry* 1987; **144**: 1403–11.

5. Relapse prevention

Relapse prevention is the primary focus of the maintenance phase of treatment. The maintenance phase begins after a period of sustained clinical remission (8 or more consecutive weeks with 2 or fewer moderate symptoms) because, at this point, the treatment objectives shift from those related to resolving the symptoms of the last acute episode to maximizing the patient's quality of life by preventing recurrences. A summary of initial clinical decision points for relapse prevention is shown in Figure 10.

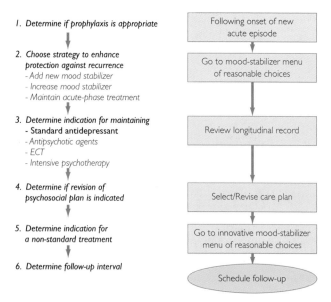

Figure 10 *Initial clinical decision points for relapse prevention.*

The available literature provides valuable, albeit incomplete, guidance to the clinician attempting to match individual bipolar patients with prophylactic treatment strategies. Although the literature is a good starting point, the process of sustaining remission and maximizing quality of life is best guided by careful assessment of the individual's response to treatment over the course of several years. When the outcome of each intervention is carefully documented, the medical record can guide the iterative development of an individualized treatment plan. A careful review of the patient's history is the best way to determine the most appropriate regimen for prophylaxis but can only be as good as the reliability of the historical information it contains. Systematic record-keeping and collection of the patient's daily mood charts greatly enhances the value of the medical record.

The maintenance phase can be divided into two parts: an early initiation phase and a later monitoring phase. During initiation, the clinical decisions relate to who to treat with what treatment regime. In the monitoring phase, follow-up care is provided to direct the routine management of the therapeutic regime, detect potential impending episodes and make interventions to sustain remission.

Treatment

Who should have maintenance treatment?

This question generates considerable unnecessary debate. Many experts recommend offering maintenance treatment to all patients who have suffered even a single acute manic episode, while others feel it is appropriate to reserve long-term maintenance treatment for patients who have experienced two or more manic episodes. Experts of the former opinion point out the 95% lifetime risk of recurrence and studies showing loss of acute and prophylactic benefit (at least of lithium) among patients with as few as three episodes. Experts of the latter opinion point out that the median duration of remission following the first acute episode is more than 4 years and the paucity of evidence justifying chronic treatment for bipolar patients beyond the first 32 weeks of recovery. Another aspect of selecting patients for maintenance treatment relates to the likelihood that patients will discontinue treatment regardless of the psychiatrist's recommendations. Patients who discontinue lithium treatment, particularly when discontinuation is abrupt, appear to be at increased risk for recurrence. Guy Goodwin and colleagues have attempted to quantify the risks and benefits of lithium maintenance and recommend against offering maintenance treatment to patients who are judged unlikely or unwilling to adhere to treatment for at least 2 years. It is unclear when patients become liable to such discontinuation phenomena or whether a similar phenomenon develops upon discontinuation of other maintenance treatments. In a large prospective study, Bowden and colleagues found no evidence of discontinuation phenomena following discontinuation of acute treatment with lithium or divalproex.

While current literature does not resolve the issue of who should have treatment, from a practical point of view the question itself is rarely of any real clinical significance. First, by the time most patients receive a bipolar diagnosis they have already suffered multiple episodes. There is no disagreement about recommending long-term maintenance therapy for bipolar patients who have experienced three or more episodes. Second, since many clinical experts recommend continuation of effective acute-phase treatments for a period of 1 year after the onset of clinical remission, a substantial proportion of bipolar patients will relapse within the period of prudent continuation treatment. Third, a surprisingly large proportion of patients simply never achieve the period of sustained euthymia considered a sufficient prerequisite to consideration of treatment discontinuation. Thus two distinct subgroups exist among the population of patients receiving long-term care: those who have achieved a stable remission and those who have not.

For those patients who attain full recovery after a first manic or hypomanic episode, it is likely to be more productive to stress the importance of maintaining treatment throughout the period of highest risk, namely, the first 32 weeks following remission, than soliciting a lifetime commitment to prophylactic treatment.

Initiation of maintenance-phase treatment

Expert guidelines (APA, 1994; Frances *et al*, 1996) support the use of 'mood stabilizers' for bipolar patients (Figures 11 and 12). For most clinicians this term came to be understood as a short-hand reference to lithium, carbamazepine and divalproex. As new medications enter the therapeutic market, there is a tendency to

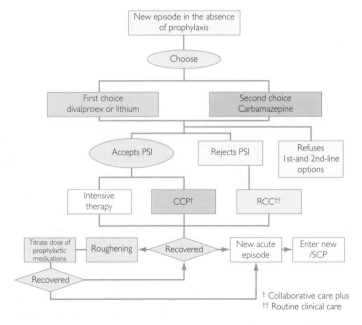

Figure 11 *The relapse prevention pathway: flowchart of treatment of patient experiencing new episode in the absence of prophylaxis.*

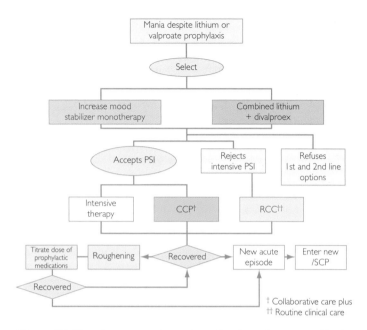

Figure 12 *The relapse prevention pathway: flowchart of treatment of patient experiencing new episode of mania despite lithium or valproate prophylaxis.*

consider medications with anticonvulsant or putative antimanic properties as 'mood stabilizers' despite the absence of any data. Figure 13 shows the mood stabilizer menu of reasonable choices.

When selecting agents it is important to be aware of the regulatory approval given to lithium and divalproex in the US and lithium and carbamazepine in Europe. Such approval reflects the ample quantity of high-quality data supporting their efficacy for at least one indication related to bipolar illness, and clearly separates them from other less-well-studied agents. Expert guidelines recommend reserving the use of novel agents to those cases with unsatisfactory response to trials of proven treatments alone and in combination. Since many bipolar patients will have an inadequate response to the well-studied therapies, knowledge of other putative and innovative treatment modalities is useful.

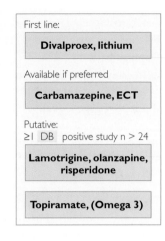

- Efficacy for ≥1
  - Acute mania
  - Acute depression
  - Mania prophylaxis
  - Depression prophylaxis
- No acute worsening
- No increase in cycling

Risk:
Intolerable adverse effects
Low (risk <0.5%)
- **Likely adverse effects:**
  Reasonably tolerable
- No specific contraindication

First line:

| **Divalproex, lithium** |

Available if preferred

| **Carbamazepine, ECT** |

Putative:
≥1 DB positive study n > 24

| **Lamotrigine, olanzapine, risperidone** |

| **Topiramate, (Omega 3)** |

Figure 13 *Mood stabilizer menu of reasonable choices.*

The treatment plan for the maintenance phase should take into account the many factors that have been implicated in triggering recurrences. Expert recommendations recognize both the essential role of 'mood-stabilizing' medications and the benefit of psychosocial interventions (including formal psychotherapies, patient/family education and self-help groups) in treatment plans aimed at relapse prevention.

Paradoxically, the first decision point in relapse prevention typically occurs during the acute phase. Somatic therapies that will comprise maintenance-phase treatment are usually initiated during the acute phase of treatment. Since the choice of acute-phase treatment strategies is often influenced by the goal of enhanced protection against recurrence, the first maintenance-phase decision point actually occurs in the acute phase. In other words, during the acute phase of mixed, manic or depressive episodes, treatment strategies are implemented that lay the foundation for relapse prevention. Sometimes, as in the case of a patient with breakthrough mania during lithium prophylaxis, the addition of divalproex targets prophylaxis as well as acute symptoms. Similarly, the strategy of discontinuing standard antidepressant medication during a manic episode may be chosen with the aim of minimizing future recurrences. In other circumstances, as when attempts to taper antipsychotics or antidepressants are followed by relapse, historical evidence indicates incorporating the successful acute-phase therapies into the maintenance regime.

Determining the most appropriate regimen for prophylaxis

At the conclusion of the acute and continuation phases, the patient's treatment regime is reviewed to determine which of the variety of therapies is to be used as maintenance phase-treatment and which will be discontinued. As yet, no controlled data exist to answer questions concerning differential response to various prophylactic medications. Nor is there data to inform the choice of strategies for patients who have experienced breakthrough episodes. Determination of which therapies are most appropriate to include in an individual's prophylactic regime should be based on a careful review of that patient's history.

Treatments other than those that are currently considered 'mood stabilizers' may well be appropriate for some patients. Generally, however, it is prudent to consider a gradual taper of acute-phase medications, such as standard antidepressants and antipsychotics. Treatment with antidepressants has been associated with increased cycle frequency and the induction of rapid cycling. Conventional or 'typical' neuroleptics have often been used during the maintenance phase, despite concern about tardive dyskinesia and data showing that maintenance treatment with flupenthixol resulted in more frequent depressions than maintenance with placebo. Atypical antipsychotics show advantages over typical antipsychotics in terms of safety, including low incidence of tardive dyskinesia. There is as yet no double-blind controlled data for atypical antipsychotic medications. Suppes reported better outcomes among bipolar patients, however, when clozapine was included in the regimen of bipolar patients than those maintained on treatment excluding clozapine. Case reports have raised concern that atypical antipsychotics can induce mania, but this phenomenon has not been observed in prospective studies.

Special populations for maintainence-phase treatment

Breakthrough episodes during taper
Patients suffering relapse during the course of taper may be appropriate candidates for chronic treatment with antipsychotic or antidepressant medications.

Breakthrough episodes on mood-stabilizer monotherapy
Patients experiencing a recurrence despite therapeutic levels of lithium. Carbamazepine or divalproex are candidates for either combination mood-stabilizer maintenance therapy or maintenance with the mood-stabilizer monotherapy at an increased dose.

Following mixed episodes
Since the treatment recommendations for patients with mixed episodes are the same as those in the mania pathway, most patients with mixed episodes will have tapered their antidepressant medication. Data from the NIMH collaborative study suggest that maintaining treatment with standard antidepressants following resolution of mixed episodes is particularly risky. Antidepressants may, however, have been reintroduced for those patients with persistent depression following resolution of the manic component of the mixed episode. In such cases, a slow taper of standard antidepressant is recommended following an appropriate continuation phase.

Following ECT

Patients responding to acute treatment with ECT can be sub-grouped according to whether ECT was used as a matter of choice (e.g. symptom acuity warranted aggressive treatment) or because the acute episode proved refractory to other somatic interventions. In either case, early relapse is common following abrupt discontinuation of ECT. In all cases, mood-stabilizing medications should be offered for prophylaxis and, in the latter case, consideration should be given to the use of continuation ECT as a preventative treatment.

Women seeking to conceive

Bipolar illness is not an absolute contraindication to child-bearing. When women with bipolar disorders and their spouses seek counseling prior to conception, a review of the teratogenic potential of the treatment is necessary as well as the risk of relapse during gestation and the postpartum period. Generally, most experts recommend delaying attempts to conceive until patients have enjoyed a stable remission for at least 6–12 months. Selection of treatment strategy for women with bipolar disorders with stable remission should take into account the severity and frequency of prior episodes, age of the patient, and the quality of available supports. A range of management options should be reviewed, allowing individual patients and their partners to choose the risks most acceptable. Older women or those with more severe episodes may choose to conceive while maintaining treatment and use fetal ultrasound or amniocentesis to screen for potential teratogenic effects. Younger women and those with milder illness may more reasonably plan to taper some or all medication prior to conception, while relying on non-pharmacologic strategies at least through the first trimester. Consultation with psychopharmacologists, gynecologists, teratologists or pediatricians familiar with the issues is often valuable.

Women who have become pregnant during the course of maintenance treatment

Management depends largely on when in the course of gestation pregnancy is recognized, and which medications are in use. As above, patient preference is the key determinant in selecting treatment strategies. In view of teratogenicity, the choice of rapid discontinuation becomes progressively less appealing as the pregnancy progresses beyond the first 10 weeks. When this option is chosen, tapering over a 1–2 week period may reduce the risk of early relapse without substantially altering the risk of teratogenicity, but plans should be made in advance for intervention in the event of relapse and close follow-up offered.

Determining the appropriate psychosocial intervention

Specialized versions of psychosocial interventions such as family-focused therapy, interpersonal social rhythms therapy, life goals and cognitive behavioral therapy, have shown promise as adjunctive interventions in the maintenance phase of treatment.

Even where these specific treatments are not readily available it seems wise to incorporate the common elements of these good mood hygiene interventions into the treatment plan to whatever extent is feasible. The Collaborative Care Model developed at the Massachusetts General Hospital (MGH) recommends that patients use these elements to develop an individualized written management plan that does not rely entirely on the patient for executive function. Samples and directions for constructing treatment contracts can be accessed via the internet (www.manicdepressive.org).

Monitoring visit interval

There are no empirical data to guide the choice of interval between monitoring visits. Even within national boundaries, practice varies widely across geographic regions and treatment settings. The Collaborative Care Model offers a flexible approach to monitoring intervals. In this model the default recommendation is for monthly monitoring visits throughout the remainder of 1 year following the end of the acute phase. Over the next year, patients remaining well are seen every other month. After 2 years in remission patients are seen quarterly.

Monitoring continuation-phase treatment

Once a stable treatment regime has been established, routine follow-up visits focus on four main tasks: maintaining prophylactic treatments within the therapeutic range, managing comorbid conditions, managing adverse effects, and monitoring for impending episodes.

Maintaining prophylactic treatments within the target range

Although the boundaries of the therapeutic range for lithium (0.5–1.0 mmol/l), divalproex (50–120 μg/ml) and carbamazepine (4–12 μg/ml) rest more on clinical tradition than empirical data, available data is generally consistent with the ideas that most patients will experience therapeutic benefit when above the lower limit and few will benefit only at levels above the upper limit. For clinical purposes, it is important to recognize that maintaining serum levels in the therapeutic range presents a broad and sometimes shifting clinical goal. During the transition from the acute phase to the maintenance phase it is often necessary to adjust dosage of mood-stabilizing medications. Tolerance of adverse effects generally decreases when acute manic symptoms resolve and, at least in the case of lithium and carbamazepine, serum levels may change.

Managing comorbid conditions

It is unusual to meet bipolar patients who do not have comorbid conditions. Psychiatric comorbidity that is especially common among bipolar patients includes anxiety disorders, alcohol and substance abuse, as well as attention-deficit and other disruptive behavior disorders of childhood. The national comorbidity study makes it clear that comorbidity is a signficant risk factor predictive of relapse. Although representing only 14% of subjects with any diagnosis, the subset that met DSM-IV criteria for three or more disorders accounted for 90% of the severe episodes that occurred over 1 year of follow-up.

Left untreated, these disorders contribute to dysphoria, counterproductive self-treatment and, particularly when associated with insomnia, may interfere with treatment response. In many cases, treatment of these conditions has salutary effects on the course of bipolar illness or vice versa. Unfortunately, standard treatment for some of these conditons (e.g. treatment of obsessive–compulsive disorder with selective serotonin reuptake inhibitors or stimulants for attention-deficit disorder) can exacerbate bipolar disorder.

Use of an anxiolytic agent is often warranted to ameliorate symptoms of anxiety disorders, restore sleep and to truncate excessive response to stressors. Small open trials have found that high-potency benzodiazepines such as alprazolam and clonazepam often produce a rapid benefit by significantly relieving dysphoria in some bipolar depressed patients. It remains unclear, however, whether the patients described experienced a true antidepressant effect or simply improved scores on depression rating scales as a result of diminished anxiety.

For anxious patients with contraindication to benzodiazepines or non-response to benzodiazepine, gabapentin, clonidine or propranolol may be useful adjuncts. Adrenergic blockers must be used with caution since they may contribute to depression or interfere with antidepressant medications.

For bipolar patients who experience successful resolution of the acute phase and maintain stability through the continuation phase, tapering of anxiolytic drugs is usually indicated. Some bipolar patients, however, appear to benefit from maintenance anxiolytic therapy.

Bipolar patients appear to have a particular vulnerability to substance abuse, which in turn worsens the prognosis. Reports suggest a dramatic increase in all-cause mortality and risk of suicide in untreated bipolar patients with substance abuse, making it clear that treatment for substance abuse should be a priority in the treatment of bipolar illness.

Managing adverse effects

Although spontaneous reports might suggest otherwise, nearly all bipolar patients experience adverse effects attributable to maintenance treatment. Since a substantial proportion of otherwise treatment-responsive patients discontinue treatment because of adverse effects, it is useful to actively monitor for expected adverse effects and inform the patient of the likely management. At the MGH Bipolar Clinic in Boston, the most common reasons for patients to discontinue successful treatment during the maintenance phase were weight gain, cognitive impairment, gastrointestinal complaints, and hair loss. Active management of adverse effects with patient education allows many patients to sustain beneficial treatment; this includes a willingness on the clinician's part to acknowledge the possibility that treatment is indeed causing the adverse effect and to offer alternatives. Treatment discontinuation can often be avoided by changing the amount, timing, and form of problematic medications. This is particularly true for adverse effects such as nausea and tremor, which are associated with peak drug levels.

Roughening and recurrence

Many patients experience intermittent subsyndromal symptoms (roughening) during the discontinuation/maintenance phase. Roughening may be the harbinger of an impending acute episode or merely a brief period of mild symptoms with little clear relation to the patient's mood disorder. Studies of such inter-episode symptoms performed by Keller and others suggest that roughening with features of depression often resolves without intervention. Symptoms of hypomania convey the risk of evolving into full affective episodes. When managing roughening, increased vigilance is usually necessary and consideration should be given to increased frequency of visits and prophylactic medication as a means of aborting a potential new acute episode.

The occurrence of symptoms meeting criteria for an acute episode would be considered a recurrence (new episode) requiring re-introduction of acute treatments.

Endpoint

The main endpoint in the relapse prevention pathway involves either augmenting or interrupting the course of treatment that is aimed at relapse prevention when the patient suffers a new acute episode. Patients may enter the acute-depression pathway or the mood-elevation pathway for a course of acute treatment and re-enter the relapse-prevention pathway after achieving a stable remission. Transitions to these pathways are common for patients with bipolar illness and need not be viewed as treatment failure. When treatment returns to the relapse prevention pathway the question of altering the relapse prevention therapies should be addressed, based on whether the long-term trend indicates fewer, briefer or milder episodes.

Treatment success, even when euthymia extends over a period of years, is not itself an indication to discontinue treatment. Any decision to reduce treatments aimed at relapse prevention should be weighed in the context of potential risks and benefits.

Suggested reading

American Psychiatric Association. Practice guideline for the treatment of patients with bipolar disorder. *Am J Psychiatry* 1994; **151** (Suppl. 12): 1–35.

Basco MR, Rush AJ. *Cognitive-Behavioral Therapy for Bipolar Disorder*. The Guilford Press: New York, 1996.

Bauer MS, McBride L, Chase C *et al.* Manual-based group psychotherapy for bipolar disorder: a feasibility study. *J Clin Psychiatry* 1998; **59**: 449–55.

Bowden CL, Calabrese JR, McElroy SL *et al* for the Divalproex Maintenance Study Group. A randomized, placebo-controlled 12-month trial of divalproex and lithium in treatment of outpatients with bipolar I disorder. *Arch Gen Psychiatry* 2000; **57**: 481–9.

Coryell W, Winokur G, Solomon D *et al.* Lithium and recurrence in a long-term follow-up of bipolar affective disorder. *Psychol Med* 1997; **27**: 281–9.

Frances A, Docherty JP, Kahn DA. The expert consensus guideline series. Treatment of bipolar disorder. *J Clin Psychiatry* 1996; **57** (Suppl. 12A): 1–88.

Gelenberg AJ, Kane JM, Keller MB *et al.* Comparison of standard and low serum levels of lithium for maintenance treatment of bipolar disorder. *N Engl J Med* 1989; **321**: 1489–93.

Goodwin FK, Jamison KR. *Manic–Depressive Illness.* Oxford University Press: New York, 1990.

Greil W, Ludwig-Mayerhofer W, Erazo N. Lithium versus carbamazepine in the maintenance treatment of bipolar disorders – a randomised study. *J Affect Disord* 1997; **43**: 151–61.

Maj M, Pirozzi R, Magliano L, Bartoli L. Long-term outcome of lithium prophylaxis in bipolar disorder: a 5-year prospective study of 402 patients at a lithium clinic. *Am J Psychiatry* 1998; **155**: 30–5.

Miklowitz DJ, Goldstein MJ. *Bipolar Disorder. A Family-Focused Treatment Approach.* The Guilford Press: New York, 1997.

Priebe S, Broker M. Initial response to active drug and placebo predicts outcome of antidepressant treatment. *Eur Psychiatry* 1997; **12**: 28–33.

Prien RF, Klett CJ, Caffey EM Jr. Lithium prophylaxis in recurrent affective illness. *Am J Psychiatry* 1974; **131**: 198–203.

Prien RF, Kupfer DJ, Mansky PA *et al.* Drug therapy in the prevention of recurrences in unipolar and bipolar affective disorders. Report of the NIMH Collaborative Study Group comparing lithium carbonate, imipramine, and a lithium carbonate–imipramine combination. *Arch Gen Psychiatry* 1984; **41**: 1096–104.

Sachs GS, Thase ME. Bipolar disorder therapeutics: maintenance treatment. *Biol Psychiatry* (in press).

Solomon DA, Ryan CE, Keitner GI *et al*. A pilot study of lithium carbonate plus divalproex sodium for the continuation and maintenance treatment of patients with bipolar I disorder. *J Clin Psychiatry* 1997; **58**: 95–9.

Suppes T, Baldessarini RJ, Faedda GL *et al*. Discontinuation of maintenance treatment in bipolar disorder: risks and implications (review). *Harv Rev Psychiatry* 1993; **1**: 131–44.

Suppes T, Webb A, Paul B *et al*. Clinical outcome in a randomized 1-year trial of clozapine versus treatment as usual for patients with treatment-resistant illness and a history of mania. *Am J Psychiatry* 1999; **156**: 1164–9.

6. Rapid cycling

Rapid cycling, defined by the occurrence of four or more episodes or two complete cycles (two high and two low phases) in a 12-month period, is a term coined by Dunner and Feive to describe a common finding among bipolar patients with poor response to lithium.

The prevalence of rapid cycling is estimated to be 5–15% of those with bipolar disorder; most studies find a female gender predominance among rapid cycling. The female:male gender ratio ranges from 2:1 to 9:1. Despite some inconsistency between studies, hypothyroidism is considered a strong risk factor. Studies of cycle frequency find that its distribution is skewed toward higher frequency cycling although it can be difficult to evaluate patients with brief cycle lengths. There is no reliable way to differentiate ultrarapid cycling (cycle length <24–48 hrs) from mixed episodes, nor is there a clinical reason to approach the treatment of these conditions differently.

The DSM-IV designates rapid cycling as a course specifier rather than a distinct subtype of bipolar illness. The vast majority of bipolar patients who experience a period of rapid cycling during the course of their illness will also experience periods without rapid cycling. Rapid cycling over periods of years appears to be the exception rather than the rule. Patients with sustained rapid cycling should be carefully evaluated for possible substance abuse and other medical conditions, which might account for the pattern of sustained rapid cycling (e.g. medications, multiple sclerosis, head injury, mental retardation and EEG abnormalities).

Treatment

Initiating treatment

Treatment for rapid cycling is by definition aimed at reducing cycle frequency and might be considered as a special instance of relapse prevention. While true in the abstract, the clinical reality is somewhat paradoxical. Patients with rapid cycling typically present with varying degrees of acute symptomatology and fluctuating polarity. The difference between the treatment of rapid and nonrapid cycling patients is the management of acute phase symptomatology rather than the continuation or maintenance-phase management. The criteria for entering the rapid cycling pathway is that the patient's current clinical status is compatible with avoiding or tapering standard antidepressants or other cycle promoting agents.

The first step in treatment directed against cycling should be to establish a mood-stabilizing regime that eliminates cycle promoting agents and adds or optimizes medications with mood-stabilizing properties. In practice this most often means tapering off antidepressant medications, steroids, sympathomimetics and stimulants (including caffeine) (Figure 14). Consideration should be given to eliminating any other agents that have been implicated as cycle promoting or inducing mania (e.g. DHEA, bronchodilators, gonadotropins, oral contraceptives, muscle relaxants and triazolobenzodiazepines). Reports from Kukopulos and Wehr suggest that iatrogenic factors frequently fuel rapid cycling. Therefore, although not a designation in the DSM, it can be useful to classify rapid cycling as primary or secondary.

Considerations for special subpopulations

Primary rapid cycling

Primary rapid cycling describes persistent recurrence over at least four months in the absence of antidepressant medications, other substances or a general medical condition that is associated with the induction of mania or promoting cycling. Primary

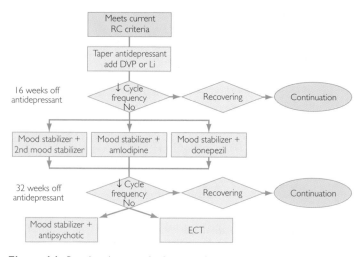

Figure 14 *Rapid cycling: standard care pathway.*

rapid cycling is frequently difficult to treat and can be made worse by cycle-promoting agents.

Secondary rapid cycling
Secondary rapid cycling refers to instances where a secondary factor is believed to play an etiological role in sustaining a rate of cycling which otherwise would be less than 4 per year. In most such cases, the bipolar disorder is correctly diagnosed as a primary mood disorder but the pattern of rapid cycling is secondary (substance induced or due to a general medical condition). Secondary rapid cycling is often responsive to elimination or amelioration of factors that might destabilize mood or promote cycling (Table 7). Some bipolar patients with apparent secondary rapid cycling become intensely dysphoric or even euphoric soon after tapering standard antidepressant medication. These patients can be managed by shifting to acute-phase management and, after again achieving remission, resuming taper on a more gradual schedule.

Table 7 *Summary of common decision points in rapid cycling.*

Decision point	Suggested starting point
Determine need for acute-phase antidepressant treatment	Review current symptom acuity and cycle frequency over past 4 episodes.
Identify possible secondary factors	Look for hypothyroidism or substance abuse
Taper any antidepressants	20–33% per month
Optimize/Add anticycling agents	Lithium or divalproex if not already present
Evaluate outcome	Use systematic assessment and prospective charting
Add additional anticycling agent(s)	See menu of putative mood stabilizing agents (see Figure 9)
When to shift priority to management of acute episode	Evaluate safety and patient tolerance

Treatment for comorbid condition as putative cause of secondary rapid cycling

Treatment for comorbid condition is a putative cause of secondary rapid cycling, particularly for patients with comorbid conditions such as OCD, panic, bulimia or ADHD. Where the preferred treatments for a comorbid condition may fuel rapid cycling, the preferable option is to attempt to treat the comorbid condition by maximizing or adding a mood stabilizer. Several medications classified as putative mood stabilizers have been shown to have a salutary effect on one or more common comorbid conditions. When this proves unsuccessful, alternative treatment for the comorbid condition without cycle-promoting properties should be attempted (e.g. clonidine for ADHD). If a third intervention is required (e.g. severe comorbid OCD responsive only to SSRI), minimizing the dose of the offending agent to a level just sufficient to allow treatment with cognitive behavior therapy offers a compromise between conflicting treatment objectives.

Common decision points

Determine appropriate acute-phase treatment

Treatment for acute mania generally does not conflict with treatment for rapid cycling. Occasional case reports, which have implicated phenothiazines as cycle-promoting agents in individual cases, make avoiding these agents worthy of consideration.

Treatment for depression is much more problematic. As a rule the deciding factor in prescribing antidepressants to rapid cycling patients is the patient's ability to tolerate and safely endure periods of dysphoria. At any time that patient–doctor judgment deems it appropriate, the care of rapid cycling patients can be shifted to the approach usual for acute bipolar depression and standard antidepressant medications can be judiciously administered. There are, however, circumstances where the use of antidepressants can be discouraged as imprudent. For example, standard antidepressant medications are unlikely to benefit patients with a history of dysphoria lasting less than 2 weeks, or those for whom prior treatment trials demonstrate a duration of remission shorter than 4 weeks despite continued treatment with standard antidepressants.

In the many instances in which patients are willing to abstain from standard antidepressants, the primary objective of acute treatment becomes maintaining safety while implementing interventions that can relieve the dysphoria without adversely affecting the course of the illness. Such interventions are by definition mood stabilizers and may include lithium, anticonvulsants, atypical antipsychotics, cholinesterase inhibitors (donepezil) as well as psychosocial interventions.

Optimize/Add anticycling agents

Selection of mood stabilizer

There are few controlled prospective studies of rapid cycling. Patients with rapid cycling respond less well to lithium than non-rapid cycling patients. To generalize from this observation that lithium is not beneficial for rapid cycling is misleading. Clearcut nonresponse to lithium is observed only when response is defined narrowly as having no recurrence at all. The available literature does, however, indicate a consistent benefit of lithium in reducing cycle frequency. Given the refractory nature of rapid cycling, all putative mood stabilizing medications and antimanic agents may be considered rational options for treatment of rapid cycling, but preference should be given to agents with established mood stabilizing or antimanic efficacy.

Although there is no prospective comparative data, uncontrolled reports of good treatment response to anticonvulsant medications such as divalproex or carbamazepine in patients with a history of rapid cycling and nonresponse to lithium have established these agents as preferable to lithium as initial treatment for rapid cycling. As illustrated in Figure 14 the recommended pathway starts with two interventions, tapering any antidepressants and adding either divalproex or lithium.

Several reports indicate that some patients refractory to first-line mood stabilizers may respond well to a wide array of treatments including atypical antipsychotic medications (clozapine, risperidone, olanzapine or quetiapine), other anticonvulsants (lamotrigine, gabapentin or topiramate), thyroxine, calcium channel blockers, cholinomimetics (donepezil or choline), Omega-3 fatty acids, bright light and ECT. Psychosocial interventions may be beneficial in ameliorating depression and reducing recurrence of depression. Several promising psychosocial interventions developed specifically for bipolar illness target reducing interpersonal conflict, management of potential episode triggers and/or stabilizing circadian rhythms.

Evaluating outcome
In evaluating the impact of each anticycling intervention, mere resolution of a current acute episode in itself should not be considered evidence of improvement nor should any single recur-

rence be taken as treatment failure. Prospective mood charts can help guide treatment decision making, especially if they provide clear evidence of fewer, briefer or milder episodes. Even in the face of intermittent periods of severe depression and/or mania, evidence of decreased cycle frequency over the first 3 months of taper is often the harbinger of progressive improvement. The benefit of adding a new mood stabilizer or discontinuing anti-depressants may not be apparent for several months. Thus, in assessing the outcome of interventions in this pathway, little confidence can be given to presumed effects observed over time periods less than 3 cycle lengths or 4 months. For some interventions evidence of efficacy may require sustained treatment over 6 months or longer.

Add additional anticycling agent(s)

Clinical imperatives make it unreasonable to delay adding new interventions for periods longer than 4 months. Titration of each intervention to an individual's optimal dose is an art greatly aided by thoughtful review of a daily mood chart (see Appendix A). Upward titration to maximal dose of each mood stabilizer is a reasonable option limited by the tolerability of each agent. After three cycle lengths or six months at a given dose, agents with no apparent benefit may be tapered off. Patients with partial benefit may be given additional time on the current regime or additional agents can be added.

Patients remain in the rapid cycling pathway until treatment achieves a stable remission, which in theory would allow management of acute depressive episodes in the same manner as nonrapid cycling patients. Logically this judgment implies rapid cycling has been broken but there is no data to determine if in fact absence of the rapid cycling state indicates a transition to a less pernicious disease state or a simple lack of overt expression of an enduring trait. With this caution, a suggested minimal criterion for exiting the rapid cycling pathway when well requires a stable recovery for at least 1 year.

Consequently, the long-term management of the majority of rapid cycling patients remains in the rapid cycling pathway even though their rate of recurrence no longer meets the criteria for rapid cycling. The major focus for patients experiencing 1–3 episodes per year is to use the iterative treatment/assessment process to progressively improve their overall regime aiming at the highest possible quality of life. The maintenance of records documenting incremental improvement over the span of years is an invaluable asset for maintaining the therapeutic optimism of patient, family and clinician as well as guiding the next therapeutic trial.

Endpoints

The main endpoints in the rapid cycling pathway involve either interrupting the course of treatment aimed at rapid cycling in order to treat intolerable acute symptoms or declaring the patient recovered from rapid cycling.

When the patient suffers an acute episode that requires treatment with standard antidepressant medications, the therapeutic focus shifts from rapid cycling to standard management of acute bipolar depression (see Chapter 4). Patients may also require management in accordance with the acute mania pathway (see Chapter 3). Transitions to these pathways are common over the course of bipolar illness. When the acute symptoms remit, treatment returns to the rapid cycling pathway.

Patients meeting remission criteria for more than 1 year are candidates for transition to the standard relapse prevention pathway (see Chapter 5). Clinicians and patients should be aware that leaving the more restrictive guidelines of this pathway carries with it an as yet unsubstantiated assumption that rapid cycling represents a state rather than a trait. When selecting treatment for the next new episode, even a distant history of rapid cycling should be taken into account.

Common triggers for affective instability are listed in Table 8.

Table 8 *Common triggers for affective instability.*

Sleep loss
Alcohol/Substance abuse or withdrawal
EEG abnormality
Hypothyroidism
Migraine headache
Nicotine withdrawal
Rapid discontinuation of lithium

Antidepressants
   Use
   Discontinuation

Other medications
   Steroids
      Anabolic steroids
      Glucocorticoids
   Sympathomimetics
      Stimulants, caffeine, decongestants, bronchodilators, anorectics
   Reproductive hormones/blockers
      Gonadotropins
      Oral contraceptives
      Testosterone
      DHEA
      Lupron
      Clomid
   Muscle relaxants
   Triazolobenzodiazepines
   Treatment for Parkinson's disease
   Thyroxine
   Barbiturates

Interpersonal
   Conflict/Trauma
   Grief
   Success
   Loss of support systems

Circadian disruptions
   Seasonality
   East–west Travel
   Shift work

Suggested reading

Akiskal HS. The prevalent clinical spectrum of bipolar disorders: Beyond DSM-IV. *J Clin Psychopharmacol* 1996; **16** (Suppl. 1), 4S–14S.

Bauer MS, Whybrow PC. Rapid cycling bipolar affective disorder. II. Treatment of refractory rapid cycling with high-dose levothyroxine: a preliminary study. *Arch Gen Psychiatry* 1990; **47**: 435–40.

Bowden CL, Calabrase JR, McElroy SL *et al.* The efficacy of lamotrigine in rapid cycling and non-rapid cycling patients with bipolar disorder. *Biol Psychiatry* 1999; **45**: 953–8.

Calabrese JR, Delucchi GA: Spectrum of efficacy of valproate in 55 patients with rapid-cycling bipolar disorder. *Am J Psychiatry* 1990; **147**: 431–4.

Kusumakar V, Yatham LN, Haslam DRS *et al.* Treatment of mania, mixed state and rapid cycling. *Can J Psychiatry* 1997; **42** (Suppl. 2): 79S–86S.

Wehr T, Goodwin FK. Tricyclics modulate frequency of mood cycles. *Chronobiologia* 1979; **6**: 377–85.

Wehr T, Sack D, Rosenthal N *et al.* Rapid cycling affective disorder: contributing factors and treatment responses in 51 patients. *Am J Psychiatry* 1998; **145:** 179–84.

7. Antidepressant practical pharmacology

The antidepressants are a heterogeneous group of compounds linked by the capacity to relieve the signs and symptoms of depression. Conceptually, all currently available antidepressants affect the regulation of monoamine neurotransmission, principally noradrenergic and/or serotoninergic systems (Table 9). As described in Chapter 4, antidepressant treatment of bipolar depressive episodes conveys some risk of provoking manic or mixed episodes and can increase the likelihood of rapid cycling. Also, the long-term benefit of maintenance antidepressant treatment in combination with a mood stabilizer has not been established in bipolar disorder. Nevertheless, antidepressants continue to provide an important therapeutic option for the depressed bipolar patient, particularly when simpler strategies, such as monotherapy with a mood stabilizer, have not been effective. This chapter describes the pharmacology of the major classes and types of antidepressants.

Antidepressant medications can be grouped according to structure, mechanism of action, and sequence of introduction for clinical use in the US. The pharmacology of these medications will be reviewed in the order of their relevance to the contemporary management of bipolar depression.

Selective serotonin reuptake inhibitors

Selective serotonin reuptake inhibitors (SSRIs) are currently the most widely prescribed antidepressants in the US, Canada and

Table 9 Pharmacologic profile*: Tricyclic antidepressants (TCAs) versus newer antidepressant drugs.

	TCAs†	SSRIs	Bupropion‡	Venlafaxine	Nefazodone	Mirtazapine
Uptake inhibition						
Norepinephrine	✔		✔	✔		
Serotonin	±	✔		✔	±	
Dopamine			±		±	
Receptor affinities						
Dopamine (D₂)	✔¶					
Muscarinic	✔					
H₁-Histaminergic	✔					✔
Adrenergic α₁	✔				✔	
α₂						✔
Serotoninergic						
5-HT₂					✔	✔✔
5-HT₃						✔

*± Weak or intermediate efficacy; ✔ strong effect; SSRI, selective serotonin reuptake inhibitor

†Norepinephrine and serotonin reuptake inhibition vary among tricyclic antidepressants (TCAs); desipramine and nortriptyline have little effect on serotonin reuptake and only clomipramine has a sufficiently potent serotonin reuptake effect to treat obsessive–compulsive disorder

‡One or more metabolites of bupropion may have more pronounced inhibitory effects

¶Only amoxapine has proven antipsychotic effects

Europe. In the US there are five approved SSRIs: fluoxetine[1] (Prozac®), sertraline (Zoloft®), paroxetine (Paxil®), fluvoxamine (Luvox®) and citalopram (Celexa®). These compounds have different, unrelated chemical structures and are grouped together because of a common action, potent and relatively selective (*vis à vis* norepinephrine) blockade of the serotonin reuptake transporter. Compared with the tricyclic antidepressants (TCAs), the SSRIs all have a relative lack of effect on postsynaptic cholinergic, histaminergic and α_1 adrenergic receptors (see Table 10).

The SSRIs share the following advantageous characteristics:

- They can be started at a therapeutic dosage and generally do not require more than one or two dose titration adjustments;
- They can be taken once a day;[2]
- They have a generally more favorable tolerability profile than the TCA and MAOI classes of antidepressants;
- They have a high safety margin (i.e. therapeutic index) in overdose;
- They may have a lower incidence of provoking mania than the TCAs.

Importantly, the SSRIs have little effect on cardiac conduction or blood pressure. The basic pharmacologic characteristics of these five medications are summarized in Table 10.

The principal side-effects of the SSRIs include headache, gastrointestinal symptoms (nausea, cramping and/or diarrhea), insomnia, and sexual dysfunction (a reduction of libido and delayed ejaculation or inability to achieve orgasm). The SSRIs can cause both sedation and anxiety/agitation. Although most people treated

---

[1] Fluvoxamine has received approval from the United States Food and Drug Administration (FDA) for treatment of obsessive compulsive disorder, but not depression. It is available widely outside the US as an antidepressant.

[2] A divided dose of fluvoxamine is recommended by the manufacturer at doses of above 100 mg/day, although single daily dosing is usually feasible.

Table 10 *Comparative pharmacokinetic properties of selective serotonin re-uptake inhibitors (SSRIs).*

Typical Dose	Fluoxetine 10–60	Paroxetine 20–50	Sertraline 50–200	Fluvoxamine 50–300	Citalopram 20–60
Active metabolites	Norfluoxetine	None	N-desmethyl-sertraline*	None	None
Elimination half-life					
Parent drug	2–3 days	21 hours	26 hours	15 hours	35 hours
Active metabolite	7–9 days	—	2–4 days	—	—
Time to steady state	30–60 days	4–5 days	4–5 days	3 days	7–8 days
Linearity	Non-linear	Non-linear	Linear	Non-linear	Linear
Protein binding (%)	>95	>95	>95	~77	~80
Age effect†	Yes	Yes	Yes	No	No
Hepatic disease‡	x3	x1.8	x2	x1.6	x2
Renal disease‡	No	No	x1.5	No	No

*Activity of metabolite is markedly lower than that of parent compound
†Increased levels in elderly
‡Increased levels (x2 = two-fold elevation)

77

with SSRIs report improved sleep, effects on sleep architecture include suppression of rapid eye movement sleep, increased nocturnal awakenings, and a reduction of sleep efficiency. Uncommon but clinically important side-effects include bradycardia and the syndrome of inappropriate secretion of antidiuretic hormone (SIADH). A syndrome resembling akathisia with accompanying suicidal ideation also has been described, although there is no evidence that the risk of this adverse outcome is greater with the SSRIs than with other antidepressants. Moreover, the risk of suicide is greater in untreated depression than during SSRI therapy.

Although the SSRIs are more alike than different, there are some meaningful differences among this group of medications. For example, people who fail to respond to or tolerate one SSRI often do well when switched to another 'classmate'. The five drugs differ markedly in elimination half-lives. This has several implications: for example, the SSRIs with shorter half-lives must be discontinued for 7–10 days before beginning a monoamine oxidase inhibitor (MAOI), whereas a 28–35-day washout must be undertaken before switching from fluoxetine to an MAOI. The long elimination half-lives of fluoxetine and its active metabolite norfluoxetine convey protection against the SSRI discontinuation syndrome, which is characterized by gastrointestinal symptoms, parasthesias, lightheadedness, insomnia and mood changes. Discontinuation syndromes are most likely after abruptly stopping paroxetine, although abrupt cessation of fluvoxamine, sertraline and citalopram also can cause this problem. Another important difference pertains to effects on sexual function. Both clinical studies and laboratory experiments suggest that the likelihood of sexual dysfunction during SSRI therapy varies across the class, ranging from fluvoxamine (the least likely) to paroxetine (the most likely).

The SSRIs also can be ranked with respect to inhibitory effects on the various hepatic cytochrome (CYP) P_{450} isoenzymes (Table 11). Of greatest relevance to the treatment of bipolar disorder are the inhibitory effects of fluvoxamine on CYP P$_{450}$ IA2, which metabolizes haloperidol, amitriptyline, imipramine and clozapine,

Table 11 *Interactions between selected newer antidepressants and substrates of the cytochrome P$_{450}$ System.* *

Cytochrome P$_{450}$ isoenzyme	Inhibitors[†‡]	Common substrate drugs
2D6	Fluoxetine (strong) Paroxetine (strong) Bupropion (moderate) Sertraline (weak to moderate)[¶] Fluvoxamine (none to moderate)[¶] Venlafaxine (weak) Citalopram (weak)	Nortriptyline Desipramine Codeine Adrenergic blockers Neuroleptics SSRIs Venlafaxine Anti-arrhythmics
3A3/4	Nefazodone (strong)□ Fluvoxamine (strong)□ Fluoxetine (moderate) Sertraline (weak)	Alprazolam Triazolam Carbamazepine Nefazodone Calcium-channel-blockers Terfenadine Astemizole Cisapride
2C19[f]	Fluvoxamine (strong) Fluoxetine (moderate) Sertraline (weak)	Diazepam Barbiturates Clomipramine Imipramine
2C9/10	Sertraline (none to weak) Fluoxetine (?)	Tolbutamide Phenytoin (s)-Warfarin
IA2	Fluvoxamine (strong)	Imipramine Amitriptyline Theophylline Propranolol Caffeine Clozapine Tacrine

For footnotes see page 80

and the effects of fluvoxamine and fluoxetine on CYP P$_{450}$ 3A3/4, which metabolizes alprazolam, triazolam, citalopram and carbamazepine. It does not appear, however, that any of the SSRIs have sufficient inhibitory effects on CYP 3A3/4 to cause serious cardiovascular interactions with terfenadine (Seldane®), astemizole (Hismanal®), or cisapride (Propulsid®). Fluoxetine and paroxetine also are potent inhibitors of CYP P$_{450}$ 2D6, which metabolizes nortriptyline, desipramine, venlafaxine, several neuroleptics and several beta-blockers. Although less potent in effects, higher doses of sertraline and citalopram also may inhibit 2D6. Across the full range of isoenzymes and effects, citalopram and sertraline have less potential for pharmacokinetic interactions than the other SSRIs.

The SSRIs do not interact pharmacokinetically with lithium salts. However, there may be some pharmacodynamic implication of several side-effects of lithium therapy, including tremor, sedation and diarrhea.

Some attention has recently been given to the secondary effects of SSRIs on reuptake of norepinephrine and dopamine as a possible mechanism for within-class differences. Specifically, paroxetine and fluoxetine are relatively more noradrenergic than citalopram and fluvoxamine, whereas sertraline has a more pronounced effect on dopamine reuptake than the other SSRIs. It remains to be seen if these pharmacologic differences have any relationship

*Adapted from Nemeroff et al. and Harvey and Preskorn
†Strong: inhibitory effect > 150%; moderate: inhibitory effect 50–150%; weak: inhibitory effect <50%.
‡: Strength of effect not established but inhibition suggested by case reports
‡ Effects of bupropion and mirtazapine have not been studied sufficiently to be included
¶ Weak or no inhibition in minimally effective clinical dosages, moderate effect in higher dosages
§ Although inhibitory effect is relatively strong, it is much lower than that of ultra-potent agents such as ketoconazole
□ Effects of paroxetine, fluvoxamine, citalopram, venlafaxine, nefazodone and mirtazapine have not been studied adequately

to treatment response or risk of mania in bipolar depression. It is plausible that such secondary pharmacologic effects may help to explain individual differences in SSRI tolerability and response.

Bupropion

Bupropion (Wellbutrin®) has a unique aminoketone structure that resembles a catecholamine. Bupropion and its four pharmacologically active metabolites have virtually no effect on serotonin reuptake and relatively weak effects on dopamine and norepinephrine reuptake. The latter effects are presumed to be the *in vivo* mechanism(s) of action. Bupropion has almost no effects on cholinergic, histaminergic or α_1 receptors.

Bupropion has a relatively short elimination half-life (Table 12) and divided daily dosing is recommended at higher therapeutic doses, even when the sustained-release formulation (Wellbutrin SR®) is prescribed. This recommendation is intended to limit peak blood levels of bupropion because there is a dose-dependent relationship between bupropion therapy and risk of seizure that becomes clinically significant at doses above 400 mg/day.

Currently, bupropion therapy is recommended not to exceed 450 mg/day. At higher doses, there is up to a 2.3–2.8% risk of seizures, which is about six times the risk associated with SSRI treatment. Use of the sustained-release formulation of bupropion, which is 'capped' at a dose of 400 mg/day is not associated with an increased risk of seizures. Nevertheless, the manufacturer recommends not using bupropion-SR for treatment of patients at higher risk of seizures, including patients with eating disorders, a history of significant head injury or epilepsy. The most common side-effects of bupropion therapy are headache, tremor, nausea, dry mouth, constipation, headache and increased sweating. This side-effect profile suggests a predominantly noradrenergic effect. Bupropion treatment also significantly reduces nicotine consumption and it is marketed for this indication in the

Table 12 Comparative pharmacokinetic properties of the newer non-SSRI antidepressants.

	Trazodone	Nefazodone	Venlafaxine	Mirtazapine	Reboxetine	Bupropion
Typical daily dose (mg)	300–600*	300–600	75–375	15–45	8–10	300–450
Active metabolite	No†	Yes†	Odesmethyl-venlafaxine	No	No	Yes
Elimination half-life						
Parent drug	4–9 hours	2–4 hours	5 hours			14 hours
Active metabolite	—	18–36 hours	11 hours		—	20–37 hours
Time to steady state	2–3 days	3–5 days	3–5 days			3–5 days
Linearity	Linear	Nonlinear	Linear			Linear
Protein binding	~90	99	27			>80
Age effect	Yes	Yes	No			No
Hepatic disease	×2	×2	×2			×1–1.5
Renal disease	No	No	×1.5–2			No
CYP P450 interactions	3†	3A3/4	2D6 (weak)	None	None	2D6

*Doses of 50–150 mg are commonly used as sedative hypnotics

†Inhibition of CYP 2D6 can result in clinically relevant levels of m-chlorophenylpiperazine, a potentially anxiogenic compound

#The effect of trazodone on the CYP450 system is not well studied but nearly 20 years of experience have not revealed any clinically significant pharmacokinetic interactions

US as Zyban®. Bupropion therapy is not associated with sexual dysfunction or weight gain, even during long-term treatment. A few patients, however, develop insomnia or agitation.

Bupropion therapy results in a moderate inhibition of CYP P$_{450}$ 2D6. This interaction can result in elevated concentrations of SSRIs, venlafaxine, desipramine, and nortriptyline when these medications are used in close sequence or in combination with bupropion.

Although bupropion is much less commonly prescribed in non-bipolar depression than the SSRIs, it shares co-equal status as a first-choice treatment for bipolar depression. Many experts consider bupropion to be particularly useful for treatment of depressions characterized by hypersomnia, weight gain, and marked anergia. There is also some evidence that bupropion may be less likely to provoke mania than a TCA. Conversely, bupropion is not widely accepted as a first-line treatment of depressions complicated by prominent anxiety, although the data in support of this practice is not compelling.

Venlafaxine

Venlafaxine (Effexor®) is not considered to be an SSRI because, at higher doses, it also inhibits reuptake of norepinephrine. This second effect results in several differences in side-effect profile and probably accounts for the increased risk of elevated blood pressure observed during treatment at higher doses. The progressively greater noradrenergic effect at higher doses also may result in an ascending dose–response relationship, resulting in a 10–15% efficacy advantage when higher-dose venlafaxine therapy is used compared with the SSRIs.

The pharmacokinetic profile of venlafaxine is characterized by a relatively short half-life and a low degree of plasma protein binding (see Table 12). The extended-release formulation of venlafaxine (Effexor®) permits once-daily dosing, at least up to 225 mg/day. Venlafaxine has an active metabolite (0-desmethylvenlafaxine), which, at steady state, is present in higher concentrations than the parent compound. Venlafaxine is a weak inhibitor of CYP P_{450} 2D6 and has little effect on other CYP P_{450} isoenzymes. Venlafaxine has been reported to inhibit the metabolism of risperidone through the 2D6 mechanism.

The side-effect profile of venlafaxine is generally comparable with the SSRIs, although there are several distinguishing characteristics. First, the incidence of nausea is greater during the first 2 weeks of therapy than observed with the SSRIs. Second, side-effects presumedly associated with noradrenergic reuptake inhibition, such as dry mouth, dizziness, appetite loss and agitation, are higher than observed with the SSRIs. Third, as noted earlier, venlafaxine treatment at doses of 150 mg/day or higher is associated with sustained elevations of blood pressure. For example, there is about a 2–3% increase of risk of elevated diastolic blood pressure (defined as an increase of at least 10 mmHg to a value above 90 mmHg at three consecutive visits) at doses of 150–225 mg/day of venlafaxine. The risk of elevated blood pressure is 8–10% among patients treated with 300–375 mg/day of venlafaxine. Fourth, venlafaxine therapy is associated with a discontinuation syndrome that is, at the least, comparable with that observed in paroxetine.

Although the extended-release formulation of venlafaxine is tolerated better than the original formulation, many psychiatrists still prefer to use venlafaxine XR as a second- or third-line therapy for bipolar depression, in other words after failure of an SSRI or bupropion. It is our experience that higher doses of venlafaxine (i.e. 225–375 mg/day) are usually necessary for such treatment-resistant cases. Blood pressure monitoring is clearly indicated when such doses are prescribed. It is not known if the risk of mania during higher-dose venlafaxine therapy is greater than observed with the SSRIs or bupropion.

Monoamine oxidase inhibitors

Three monoamine oxidase inhibitor (MAOI) antidepressants are still available for use in the USA: tranylcypromine (Parnate®), phenelzine (Nardil®), and isocarboxazid (Marplan®). These agents are described as irreversible MAOIs because they bind tightly to the enzyme. They are also referred to as **non-selective** because they inhibit both the A and B forms of MAO. Inhibition of at least 80% of MAO activity in the brain results in decreased degradative metabolism of serotonin, norepinephrine and dopamine. This is believed to be part of the mechanism of action of the MAOIs.

The irreversible and non-selective MAOIs also inhibit enzymatic activity in the gut and liver, which is necessary to metabolize tyramine and other vasoactive amines. Without deactivation, these vasoactive amines trigger paroxysmal release of norepinephrine in the sympathetic nervous system. As a result, a low tyramine diet is needed during MAOI therapy to lessen the risk of sudden and potentially dangerous hypertensive crises. All patients taking a non-selective, irreversible MAOI should be on this diet.

A fourth MAOI, selegiline (Eldepryl®) is approved for treatment of Parkinson's disease. This compound, a reversible, selective MAOI, is not an effective antidepressant at the doses approved for use by the FDA. A fifth MAOI, moclobemide (Aurorix®) is widely available outside the USA for the treatment of depression. This compound is a reversible and selective inhibitor of the MAO type A (or RIMA) and does not require the patient to be on a low tyramine diet. Unfortunately, this better tolerated MAOI does not appear to be so effective at usual antidepressant doses as the older non-selective compounds.

The MAOIs all have short half-lives and relatively simple pharmacokinetic profiles (Table 13). Divided daily dosing is generally recommended. The major concern of drug interactions pertains to their pharmacodynamic effects, particularly the potentially lethal

Table 13 Comparative profiles of the monoamine oxidase inhibitors (MAOIs).

	Isocarboxazid	Phenelzine	Tranylcypromine	Moclobemide
Typical dose (mg/day)	30–60	45–90	40–60	300–450
Substrate specificity	Non-selective	Non-selective	Non-selective	A-selective*
Enzyme binding	Irreversible	Irreversible	Irreversible	Reversible
Structure	Hydrazine	Hydrazine	Non-hydrazine	Non-hydrazine
MAOI diet	Yes	Yes	Yes	No†
Active metabolite	No	No	No	Yes
Elimination half-life	< 4 hours	< 4 hours	< 4 hours	< 4 hours
Protein binding (%)	> 95	> 95	> 95	> 95
Hepatic disease	Yes‡	Yes‡	×2	×2
Renal disease	No	No	×2	×2–3
CYP interactions¶	NA	NA	NA	NA

*Moclobemide begins to lose substrate specificity at doses above 450 mg/day

†Diet recommended at ultra-high doses

‡Hydrazine MAOIs are not recommended for patients with liver disease because of a greater risk of hepatotoxicity

¶Potential CYP$_{450}$ interactions have not been well studied. Extensive clinical experience suggests that pharmacodynamic interactions with multiple classes of drugs (e.g. TCAs, SSRIs, venlafaxine, beta-blockers, sympathomimetics and psychostimulants, and antihypertensives of all mechanisms) are much more clinically relevant

serotonin syndrome associated with concomitant exposure to an SSRI. As stated earlier, a 7–10 day wash-out period is necessary when switching from venlafaxine or an SSRI to an MAOI, with the exception of fluoxetine, for which a 28–35 day wash-out period is necessary. Seven- to 10-day wash-outs are also recommended when switching from bupropion and other antidepressants to an MAOI.

Side-effects during MAOI therapy are typically more problematic than those observed with the newer antidepressants and include orthostatic hypotension, insomnia, sedation, weight gain, edema and sexual dysfunction. However, the MAOIs do not have appreciable effects on cholinergic or histaminergic postsynaptic receptors and they can be well-tolerated by some people who cannot take 300 mg/day bupropion or 20 mg/day fluoxetine. The MAOIs also have a lower risk of cardiac toxicity than the tricyclic antidepressants, although they are still more problematic for the patient with heart disease than the SSRIs.

The need to adhere to a special diet and the relatively large average daily side-effect burden have long resulted in the use of MAOIs as second-, third-, or fourth-line therapies. Nevertheless, the MAOIs remain a valuable option for patients who cannot tolerate or do not respond to multiple other antidepressants. The MAOI tranylcypromine has a particularly strong track record for the treatment of bipolar depression, including patients who have not responded to bupropion or to SSRIs.

Other newer antidepressants

Four other antidepressants defy grouping with the medications described above: trazodone (Desyrel®), nefazodone (Serzone®), mirtazapine (Remeron®) and reboxetine (Vestra®) (see Table 12). The first three compounds are relatively sedating and share the ability to block postsynaptic 5-HT$_2$ receptors. Mirtazapine also blocks postsynaptic 5-HT$_3$ receptors and α_2 adreno- and heteroceptors. This unique combination of effects results in potentiation of norepinephrine and serotonin. Strong antihistaminic effects (roughly comparable with amitriptyline) are a principal drawback of mirtazapine.

Trazodone and nefazodone are phenylpiperazine derivatives and mirtazapine is a tetracyclic compound. None of these three drugs are potent monoamine re-uptake inhibitors and they all have a low risk of sexual dysfunction.[3] Divided daily dosing is recommended for trazodone, nefazodone and reboxetine because of relatively short half-lives. Mirtazapine can be taken once daily.

Reboxetine is a potent and selective norepinephrine reuptake inhibitor the first non-tricyclic to fit in this niche. This non-sedating compound, which is not yet approved for use in the US, has a better safety profile than the other selective norepinephrine re-uptake inhibitors, desipramine, maprotiline and nortriptyline. Its efficacy in bipolar disorder is unstudied.

Among these medications, only trazodone has significant cardiovascular toxicity, including the tendency to cause orthostasis among the elderly. Only nefazodone has a potentially significant inhibitory effect on hepatic metabolism, via CYP P_{450} 3A3/4, which can increase blood levels (and sedative effects) of alprazolam and triazolam and contraindicates use of terfenidine, astemizole and cisapride. It is not yet clear if the potent noradrenergic effects of reboxetine can increase blood pressure; this topic is receiving further study. Based on experiences with venlafaxine, this may prove to be problematic when reboxetine is added to an SSRI.

---

[3]   Priapism rarely (i.e. 6/10 000) occurs during trazodone therapy of men.

Tricyclic antidepressants and related compounds

There are ten antidepressants still available in the US that belong to this structure-based classification (Table 14). The tricyclic antidepressants (TCA) can be further subdivided into tertiary amine (amitriptyline, clomipramine, doxepin, imipramine and tri-imipramine) and secondary amine (desipramine, nortriptyline and protriptyline) groups. The remaining two compounds (amoxapine and maprotiline) are TCA derivatives.

The TCAs were the first class of antidepressants known to inhibit monoamine reuptake. The tertiary amine tricyclics inhibit reuptake of both serotonin and norepinephrine, whereas the secondary amine compounds are more selectively noradrenergic. Nevertheless, only clomipramine (Anafranil®) is sufficiently serotoninergic to treat obsessive compulsive disorder. Moreover, the active metabolites of amitriptyline and imipramine, nortriptyline and desipramine, respectively, are potent norepinephrine reuptake inhibitors. Maprotiline (Ludiomil®) is also a selective norepinephrine reuptake inhibitor.

Amoxapine (Ascendin®) is a moderately potent blocker of postsynaptic D_2 receptors, resulting in significant antipsychotic effects; however, this effect also results in the liability of extrapyramidal symptoms and the risk of tardive dyskinesia.

The TCAs and their derivatives were never ideal treatments for bipolar depression and now should be considered only when more reasonable options have failed. Beyond a plethora of side-effects attributable to blockade of anticholinergic, antihistaminic, and α_1 adrenergic receptors, the TCAs have dose-dependent effects on seizure threshold and cardiac conduction that can be lethal in overdoses as small as a 7–10-day supply of medication. The secondary amine TCAs are somewhat better tolerated and, when indicated, therapy can be guided by drug plasma levels.

Table 14 *Typical and usual maximum dosages of tricyclic antidepressants and related compounds.*

Tricyclic antidepressant drugs	Typical dose range (mg/day)	Comments
Tertiary amines		
Amitriptyline	150–250	Usual maximum: 300 mg/day
Clomipramine	100–250	Manufacturer warns not to exceed 250 mg/day
Doxepin	150–250	No longer considered less cardiotoxic than other TCAs. Maximum dose 300 mg/day
Imipramine	150–250	Usual maximum: 300 mg/day
Triimipramine	150–250	Most sedating of TCAs and possibly least potent monoamine reuptake inhibitor. Maximum dose: 300 mg/day
Secondary amines		
Desipramine	75–200	Usual maximum: 300 mg/day
Nortriptyline	50–150	Probably loss of therapeutic effect at plasma levels above 200 ng/ml
Protriptyline	30–60	Extremely long elimination half-life
Related structures		
Amoxapine	200–400	Definite antipsychotic effects
Maprotiline	150–250	Increased risk of seizures above 250 mg/day

Suggested reading

American Psychiatric Association. Practice guideline for the treatment of patients with bipolar disorder. *Am J Psychiatry* 1994; **151** (Suppl. 12): 1–35.

Frances A, Docherty JP, Kahn DA. The expert concensus guideline series. Treatment of bipolar disorder. *J Clin Psychiatry* 1996; **57** (Suppl. 12A): 1–88.

Himmelhoch JM, Thase ME, Mallinger AG, Houck P. Tranylcypromine versus imipramine in anergic bipolar depression. *Am J Psychiatry* 1991; **148**: 910–16.

Leon AC, Keller MB, Warshaw MG et al. Prospective study of fluoxetine treatment and suicidal behavior in affectively ill subjects. *Am J Psychiatry* 1999; **156**: 195–201.

Peet M. Induction of mania with selective serotonin re-uptake inhibitors and tricyclic antidepressants. *Br J Psychiatry* 1994; **164**: 549–50.

Rosenbaum JF, Fava M, Hoog SL et al. Selective serotonin reuptake inhibitor discontinuation syndrome: a randomized clinical trial. *Biol Psychiatry* 1998; **44**: 77–87.

Sachs GS, Lafer B, Stoll AL et al. A double-blind trial of bupropion versus desipramine for bipolar depression. *J Clin Psychiatry* 1994; **55**: 391–3.

Thase ME, Sachs GS. Bipolar depression: pharmacotherapy and related therapeutic strategies. *Biol Psychiatry* (in press).

Thase ME. Recent developments in the pharmacotherapy of depression. *Psychiatr Clin North Am: Ann Drug Ther* 2000; **7**: 151–71.

Thase ME, Entsuah R, Rudolph RL. Comparison of remission rates during treatment with venlafaxine or selective serotonin reuptake inhibitors: A pooled analysis of original data from 2045 depressed patients. *Br J Psychiatry* (in press).

Thase ME, Trivedi MH, Rush AJ. MAOIs in the contemporary treatment of depression. *Neuropsychopharmacology* 1995; **12**: 185–219.

8. Antipsychotic pharmacology

The antipsychotic medications have a long and checkered history as treatments for mania and psychotic bipolar depression. The antimanic effects of typical antipsychotics have been appreciated for nearly 40 years. In the largest study comparing a conventional antipsychotic and lithium, Prien and colleagues compared chlorpromazine and lithium. For those manic patients without severe motor agitation the antimanic efficacy of lithium was equivalent to chlorpromazine, and lithium was better tolerated. However for manic patients with agitation, chlorpromazine was found to have significantly greater efficacy for core symptoms such as grandiosity, motor activity, excitement, hostility and psychotic disorganization, as well as the need for ward supervision.

Given the clinical imperative to control severe symptoms in acutely manic patients, the conventional antipsychotic medications were commonly used to treat acute mania despite the considerable short-term side-effects. Conventional antipsychotics were often continued as part of maintenance treatment in the face of worry that affectively ill patients were at greater risk for tardive dyskinesia or depressive episodes than patients with schizophrenia.

These reasons form the basis of guidelines that prioritize lithium, valproate, carbamazepine and other so-called mood-stabilizing agents over conventional antipsychotics. Moreover, when conventional antipsychotics are used, guidelines often include explicit directions to minimize the dose and duration of exposure by limiting the use of conventional antipsychotics to the shortest possible duration at the lowest effective dose. This desirable aim generally led clinicians to a pattern of coprescribing antipsychotic mediations in combination with other mood stabilizers. Nevertheless, a significant minority of bipolar patients require ongoing antipsychotic therapy to remain stable.

The introduction of clozapine represented a landmark in the treatment of severe mental illness. Recognition of clozapine's potent antipsychotic effects at doses that do not cause acute extrapyramidal symptoms ushered in the era of so-called atypical antipsychotic agents. The characteristics that seem to differentiate clozapine from most conventional antipsychotic agents are relatively low potency at blocking D2 receptors and high potency of blocking $5-HT_2$ receptors. The properties are assumed to result in the 'atypical' characteristics of not causing catalepsy in animal models of antipsychotic efficacy. It is now virtually certain that clozapine treatment is associated with a low risk of tardive dyskinesia, at least within a 5 to 10 year period of observation. However, a host of serious and sometimes potentially deadly adverse effects limits the clinical utility of clozapine and has been the basis for the search for other compounds with similar pharmacological profiles. To date this search has produced three compounds that have been approved by the US Food and Drug Administration (FDA) for treatment of schizophrenia and other psychotic disorders (Table 15). These are risperidone, olanzapine and quetiapine.

Although these compounds are different in many ways, the attractive adverse effect profile of the so-called class of atypical antipsychotics has renewed interest in the use of antipsychotics as both acute-phase antimanics and putative mood stabilizers. Interestingly, reports attributing treatment emergent affective switch and exacerbation of mania to the use of atypical antipsychotics have not been confirmed in any of the controlled trials, nor have there been any convincing demonstrations of atypical antipsychotics having acute antidepressant effects when used as monotherapy or in combination with other mood stabilizers.

Table 15 *Newer (atypical) antipsychotic medications.*

Drug	US brand name	Typical daily dose (mg/day)	Common side-effects					Comments
			Sedation	Weight gain	EPS	Orthostasis	Anticholinergic	
Clozapine	Clozaril	400–650*	++++	++++	0 (+)	+++	+++	1–2% risk of agranulocytosis without WBC monitoring. Agranulocytosis rate during monitoring less than 6 per 1000. Fatality rate following agranulocytosis during monitoring is 3% (~0.8 per 10 000 exposures). Not recommended for use in combination with carbamazepine. CYP1A2 inhibitors decrease metabolism. Weak CYP2D6 inhibitor
Risperidone	Risperdal	2–6†	++	++	0 (+)	+	0	Half-life is about six times longer among CYP2D6 poor metabolizers or patients taking potent 2D6 inhibitors. This should *not* influence tolerability if dosage is titrated slowly but might affect concurrent antidepressant metabolism. Efficacy established in relation to haloperidol.

Table 15 contd.

Drug	US brand name	Typical daily dose (mg/day)	Common side-effects					Comments
			Sedation	Weight gain	EPS	Orthostasis	Anticholinergic	
Olanzapine	Zyprexa	5–15[‡]	+++	+++	0 (+)	+	++	Metabolism induced by carbamazepine and inhibited by fluvoxamine. Efficacy established in relation to haloperidol. Received FDA approval for treatment of mania in early 2000
Quetiapine	Seroquel	150–500	++	+(+)	0 (+)	++	0	Weak 2D6 inhibitor. Metabolism is slowed by potent CYP3A4 inhibitors. Divided daily dosing recommended by manufacturer. Not associated with plasma prolactin elevation at therapeutic doses. Efficacy not established in relation to haloperidol

* Remarkably slow titration is often needed i.e. initiate at 25 mg/day and increase by 25 mg units as tolerated
† Greatest D_2 receptor affinity within atypical class. Risk of EPS and prolactin elevations increase at doses above 6 mg/day. Risk of EPS is ≥2.5 times placebo at 16 mg/day
‡ Greater risk of EPS at doses above 10 mg/day. At doses ≥15 mg/day risk of EPS is ≥2.0 times placebo

The pharmacology of both the newer and older antipsychotic medications is reviewed here.

Overview of atypical antipsychotic pharmacology

Clozapine (Clozaril®)

Clozapine is a dibenzodiazepine compound and it was the first member of the class of atypical antipsychotics. There are many uncontrolled case series illustrating the utility of clozapine in bipolar disorder. Recently, Suppes *et al* (1999) found that open adjunctive treatment with clozapine produced superior outcomes over the course of 1 year's follow-up compared to adjunctive treatment with any other medication.

Clozapine is a relatively weak D_2 antagonist and a potent blocker of 5-HT$_2$, H$_1$, α_1 and muscarinic receptors. Although it is likely that clozapine has the least risk of extra-pyramidal side-effects (EPS) and tardive dyskinesia among the atypical antipsychotics, as well as an impressive ability to 'salvage' patients resistant to multiple other medications, there is a 1–2% risk of developing agranulocytosis during clozapine therapy. This potentially fatal complication necessitates fourth-line use of an otherwise highly effective medication.

Clozapine is metabolized in the liver by the CYP1A2, 2D6 and 3A4 subfamilies and its several metabolites are not therapeutically active. The 1A2 pathway is significantly inhibited by fluvoxamine, and co-therapy with this medication necessitates dosage reduction of clozapine. Although clozapine does not inhibit CYP_{450} isoenzymes, there is concern about drug–drug interactions with carbamazepine (causing bone marrow suppression), bupropion (causing increased seizure risk), benzodiazepines (causing respiratory depression) and tricyclics (giving additive anticholinergic effects and orthostasis).

Clozapine has a half-life of 11–12 hours and reaches a steady state within 3–4 days. Single daily dosing is possible, if tolerated, for some; however, for others, a divided dose is preferred. Approximately 97% of clozapine is protein bound. Blood levels of clozapine appear to be linearly proportional to doses within the therapeutic range. Dose reductions are recommended for treatment of the elderly and patients with hepatic or renal disease.

The risk of agranulocytosis during clozapine treatment peaks between the second and sixth month of therapy. Regular monitoring of the white blood count is required and therapy should be stopped if the total white cell count drops below $3000/mm^3$ or if the granulocyte count drops below $1500/mm^3$. Clozapine can be re-introduced cautiously once the granulocyte count returns to normal but must be permanently discontinued if it ever drops below $1000/mm^3$. Clozapine-induced agranulocytosis is a medical emergency and hospitalization and reverse isolation are usually necessary.

There is a 2–4% risk of seizures during clozapine therapy. This risk is greater when higher (e.g. over 600 mg/day) doses of clozapine are prescribed and when patients are taking other psychotropic drugs. Epilepsy is not an absolute contraindication for clozapine therapy, keeping in mind the potential interaction with carbamazepine. Phenytoin, also a CYP3A4 inducer, will decrease clozapine blood levels during combined treatment. In addition to fluvoxamine, antidepressants such as fluoxetine, paroxetine and nefazodone may also increase clozapine blood levels.

Other common side-effects of clozapine include sedation, hypersomnolence, sialorrhea, urinary incontinence, enuresis, weight gain, orthostatic hypotension and tachycardia. Anticholinergic side-effects (e.g. blurred vision and constipation) can also be problematic.

Risperidone (Risperdal®)
Risperdone is a benzisoxazole derivative structurally unrelated to both clozapine and the older antipsychotic medications. Study

of risperidone includes several naturalistic case series and three double-blind studies. The first (Segal *et al*, 1998), a comparison of lithium, haloperidol and risperidone for acute mania, found no difference between the treatment groups. However, the sample was too small to allow any meaningful interpretation of relative efficacy. More recently two adequately powered double-blind multicenter studies have compared combined treatment with risperidone and a mood stabilizer to placebo and mood stabilizer. In one of the studies, haloperidol and mood stabilizer were used as an active control. These studies found significant advantages in antimanic efficacy and a lower dropout rate in those patients receiving the combination of risperidone and mood stabilizer compared to those receiving mood stabilizer alone.

Risperidone is a more potent antagonist of $5-HT_2$ receptors than D_2 receptors. Early clinical trials found a rate of EPS no different than placebo. However, vigorous dosing recommendations at the time risperidone was introduced resulted in more reports of acute EPS than anticipated. Although even with such dosing risperidone is less likely to cause EPS than haloperidol, clinical experience suggests patients treated at daily doses above 4 mg can develop acute EPS.

There are insufficient comparative data to rank order the clinical significance of the dopaminergic antagonism effects of risperidone in relation to olanzapine or clozapine. Moreover, the particular doses of each compound used in studies must be examined carefully to ensure comparability. Presumably due to its effect on tuberohypophyseal dopamine receptors, risperidone is more likely than other atypical antipsychotics to cause elevation of plasma prolactin levels. However, in the absence of signs of hyperprolactinemia (e.g. amenorrhea, lactation), the clinical significance of elevated prolactin is not apparent. Risperidone is also a moderately potent antagonist of α_2 and histamine $(H)_1$ receptors.

It is likely that risperidone will prove to have a low risk of causing tardive dyskinesia. In practice, low doses (i.e. 1–4 mg/day) are much less likely to provoke EPS than high doses (i.e. 8 mg/day or more). Drawing upon experience with the older antipsychotic compounds, it is likely that the risk of tardive dyskinesia will be minimized by the use of lower doses of risperidone.

Risperidone has one active metabolite, 9-hydroxy-risperidone. Although the parent compound has a short half-life (e.g. less than 4 hours among normal metabolizers, and about 12 hours among poor metabolizers), the metabolite has a half-life of 20–22 hours and is compatible with single daily dosing in most cases. Divided daily dosing is, however, recommended for the elderly or if orthostasis is problematic. A steady state is achieved after 5–6 days of therapy.

Risperidone and its 9-OH metabolite are weak inhibitors of the CYP_{450} $2D_6$ isoenzyme. Risperidone is converted to the 9-OH metabolite by the $2D_6$ isoenzyme, although the weak $2D_6$ 'auto' inhibition does not appear to be clinically significant. 9-OH-risperidone is excreted from the kidneys and dosage adjustment is recommended for the treatment of patients with renal disease. Lower doses are similarly recommended for the treatment of the elderly.

The most common significant side-effects of risperidone therapy include EPS, weight gain and sedation. The risk of EPS is clearly dose dependent and does not differ from placebo at doses below 4 mg/day. Less than 1% of patients in clinical trials developed orthostatic hypotension. The risk of seizures in those studies was 0.3%. In acute-phase studies, 18% of patients treated with risperidone gained 7% or more of their body weight, compared with 9% of patients taking placebo. Results of several clinical trials suggest that weight gain during longer-term therapy is somewhat less with risperidone than with olanzapine therapy. Hyperprolactinemia can cause amenorrhea, decreased libido and erectile and ejaculatory dysfunction. Risperidone does not have significant effects on ECG rhythms in grouped data but occasionally patients will develop a prolongation of the Q–Tc interval.

Olanzapine (Zyprexa®)

Olanzapine is a member of the thienobenzodiazepine class of antipsychotics; it is structurally related to clozapine, the prototypic atypical antipsychotic. Case reports and open naturalistic studies found encouraging results, which led to several double-blind studies of olanzapine in mania. In two such studies the superiority of olanzapine over placebo was demonstrated. In the first study, olanzapine was initially dosed at 10 mg daily and statistical superiority was achieved in the third week. In a subsequent study, olanzapine was initially dosed at 15 mg daily and statistical superiority over placebo was achieved in the first week. These trials resulted in olanzapine's approval by the FDA for the acute-phase treatment of mania. Olanzapine has also been studied under double-blind conditions as an adjunct to mood stabilizer for acute mania. In this large study, olanzapine in combination with mood stabilizer was superior to mood stabilizer alone as early as the first week of treatment.

Olanzapine has an elimination half-life of 30 hours and steady state is achieved in 6–7 days; it can usually be taken once daily. A parenteral form of olanzapine is in development but not yet available. The drug is 93% protein bound. Olanzapine is extensively metabolized in the liver; CYP_{450} 1A2 and 2D6 are both involved in its metabolism. The metabolites of olanzapine are not known to be therapeutically active. Neither olanzapine nor its metabolites are known to inhibit CYP_{450} isoenzymes. Generally, a dosage reduction of approximately one-half is recommended for treatment of the elderly or medically compromised patient. Metabolic clearance of olanzapine is faster for men and slower for people of Asian descent and non-smokers. Individual differences in drug tolerability may be, in part, related to these factors.

The risk of seizures during olanzapine treatment is about 0.1%. Syncope resulting from orthostatic hypotension occurred in 0.6% of patients in controlled trials. Less-severe cases of postural hypotension occur more frequently (in approximately 3%); divided dosing is recommended to lessen this risk. Olanzapine does not routinely cause ECG changes besides a small incidence of tachycardia; the average heart rate increases about two beats per minute during olanzapine therapy. Prolongation of the Q–Tc interval is observed occasionally.

More common side-effects include weight gain, somnolence, fatigue, dizziness, dry mouth and constipation. More than one-half of patients taking olanzapine will gain at least 7% of their body weight during longer-term therapy. Some studies report weight gain at the rate of about 0.5 kg/wk. As with clozapine, olanzapine has been associated with alterations in insulin metabolism, and cases of treatment-emergent diabetes have been reported. Weight gain thus represents the single greatest challenge to adherence to long-term olanzapine therapy.

Olanzapine is no more likely to cause EPS at lower doses than placebo. Parkinsonian side-effects are greater at higher doses (>10 mg/day) and are about twice as common with olanzapine as with placebo. Although the risk of akathisia is low when compared with high-potency conventional neuroleptics such as haloperidol, approximately 5–10% of patients treated with olanzapine will develop this side-effect.

Quetiapine (Seroquel®)
Quetiapine is a dibenzothiazepine compound that is structurally related to clozapine and olanzapine. There are as yet no published studies of quetiapine for bipolar illness. However, case reports describe apparent antimanic efficacy. It has a short half-life (about 3 hours) and reaches steady state within 1–2 days. Divided dosing (i.e. twice daily) is usually recommended.

Quetiapine has considerably greater potency as an antagonist of postsynaptic $5HT_2$ receptors than of D_2 receptors and it does not elevate prolactin levels at therapeutic doses. Compared with the other atypical antipsychotics, quetiapine has fewer anticholinergic and antihistaminergic effects. *In vitro* studies also suggest a lower affinity for α_1 receptors, although the risk of orthostatic hypotension (discussed later in this chapter) suggests significant clinical activity.

Quetiapine is highly protein bound and shows relatively linear pharmacokinetics within the therapeutic range. Lower doses are recommended for the treatment of patients with liver or renal disease, as well as the elderly. Quetiapine is metabolized in the liver by the CYP3A4 pathway; metabolites are not therapeutically active. Carbamazepine can induce faster metabolism of quetiapine, and nefazodone, fluoxetine and fluvoxamine can inhibit its metabolism. Quetiapine is not known to have any significant effects on CYP_{450} isoenzymes.

The most commonly reported side-effects associated with quetiapine therapy are somnolence, dizziness, orthostatic hypotension and weight gain. Quetiapine is no more likely to cause EPS than placebo in low doses (i.e. 300 mg/day or less) and appears to be comparable with olanzapine at higher doses (i.e. 600–700 mg/day). Quetiapine has no significant cardiovascular effects beyond the risk of orthostasis, although again occasional cases of Q–Tc prolongation have been observed. Long-term quetiapine exposure has been associated with the development of lens opacity in dogs. Although this risk has not yet been established for humans, 'baseline' slit-lamp eye examination is recommended by the manufacturer if longer-term quetiapine therapy is contemplated.

Conventional antipsychotic medications

The conventional or typical antipsychotics can be grouped by chemical structure into six classes (Table 16):

1. Phenothiazines
2. Thioxanthenes
3. Butyrophenones
4. Dibenzoxapines

Table 16 *Older antipsychotic medications still available in the US.*

Drug	US brand name*	Typical daily dose (mg/day)	Common side-effects					Comments
			Sedation	Weight gain	EPS	Orthostasis	Anticholinergic	
Phenothiazines								
Aliphatic								
Chlorpromazine	Thorazine	300–800	++++	+++	+++	+++	++++	IM formulation not recommended for elders due to risk of orthostasis
Piperidines								
Mesoridazine	Serentil	75–300	+++	+++	++	+++	+++	Metabolite of thioridazine
Thioridazine	(Mellaril)	200–600	++++	++++	++	++++	++++	Not for use at daily doses above 800 mg. No injectable formulation. CYP2D6 inhibitor: May potentiate cardiovascular side-effects of TCAs
Piperazines								
Fluphenazine	(Prolixin)	5–20	+	+	++++	+	+	Available in decanoate formulation
Perphenazine	Trilafon	40–80	++	++	+++	++	++	CYP2D6 inhibitor
Trifluoperazine	Stelazine	20–40	++	++	++++	++	++	
Thioxanthenes								
Thiothixene	Navane*	5–40	+	+	++++	+	+	

103

Table 16 contd.

Drug	US brand name*	Typical daily dose (mg/day)	Common side-effects					Comments
			Sedation	Weight gain	EPS	Orthostasis	Anticholinergic	
Dibenzoxapines								
Loxapine	Loxitane	40–100	++	++	+++	+	+	Potent 5-HT$_{2A}$ antagonist
Butyrophenones								
Haloperidol	Haldol	5–20	+	++	++++	+	+	Available for intravenous administration. Available in decanoate formulation (dosage: 10–15 times stabilized oral daily dose) Possibly associated with greatest risk of neuroleptic malignant syndrome when high doses are instituted rapidly in combination with lithium salts
Diphenylbutylpiperidines								
Pimozide	Orap	2–10	+	+	++	0 (+)	+	FDA indication in US only for Tourette's disorder

contd

Table 16 contd.

Drug	US brand name*	Typical daily dose (mg/day)	Common side-effects					Comments
			Sedation	Weight gain	EPS	Orthostasis	Anticholinergic	
Indolones								
Molindone	Moban	40–80	++	0	++	0 (+)	+	Not available in injectable formulation

* Brand names in parantheses may only be available in the US in generic forumlations

† These are just rough guidelines for reasonably healthy adults. Smaller doses are often necessary for patients who have tolerability problems, and are usually necessary for elders and the medically frail. Higher doses are similarly indicated on occasion for treatment-resistant patients

5. Dihydroindolones
6. Diphenylbutylpiperidines

These distinctly different compounds can be grouped together as 'typical' or conventional antipsychotics because of three characteristics:

1. The capacity to cause catalepsy.
2. A relatively greater antagonism of D_2 receptors than 5-HT$_2$ receptors.
3. A relatively close correspondence between the therapeutic doses and the tendency to cause EPS.

All of the typical antipsychotics have an established risk of causing tardive dyskinesia, which may exceed 20% for patients who have had at least 3 years of antipsychotic therapy.

The phenothiazine antipsychotics include:

- The aliphatic compound chlorpromazine (Thorazine®), which was the first widely used antipsychotic
- The piperidine compound thioridazine (Mellaril®), which has the lowest potency for D_2 blockade but the greatest risk of cardiotoxicity
- The more potent piperazine subclass, consisting of trifluoperazine (Stelazine®), perphenazine (Trilafon®) and fluphenazine (Prolixin®).

Among the remaining classes, the butyrophenone haloperidol (Haldol®) is still the standard of antipsychotic potency. Thiothixene (Navane®) and loxapine (Loxitane®) are now less-commonly prescribed. The latter compound may be the closest of the conventional antipsychotics to the atypicals. Molindone (Moban®) is known primarily for a lower risk of weight gain, although we note that this potentially large benefit has not been studied extensively. Pimozide (Orap®), a diphenylbutylpiperidine, is a potent antipsychotic but it is only approved in the US for treatment of Tourette's syndrome.

All of the typical antipsychotics are highly lipid soluble and can be administered once daily; steady states are generally achieved within 4–7 days of oral dosing. All are highly protein bound. Brain drug concentrations are typically two times greater than the levels measured in the plasma. All but thioridazine and molindone have injectable formulations. Depot formulations of fluphenazine and haloperidol also are available; these formulations may take as long as 2–3 months to achieve steady state and are typically started following stabilization on oral medication.

Most of the typical antipsychotics undergo extensive hepatic metabolism, involving the CYP2D6 and, less commonly, 3A4 subfamilies. Chlorpromazine, thiothixene and thioridazine have active metabolites. In the latter case, the metabolite (mesoridazine) is also marked as an antipsychotic (Serentil®).

The clinical potency of each of the typical antipsychotic medications is almost perfectly correlated with the affinity for blockade of the D_2 receptor. Doses of 400 mg/day of chlorpromazine or 5 mg/day of haloperidol are considered minimal therapeutic doses for healthy adults (lower doses are therapeutic for the elderly); these dosages produce 60–80% D_2 receptor occupancy in the striatum and basal ganglia. The dosages of the other conventional agents can be described in terms of haloperidol or chlorpromazine equivalents. Chronic treatment with therapeutic doses of conventional antipsychotics produce a sustained reduction in the firing rate of midbrain dopamine neurons, which has been called depolarization inactivation. The fact that atypical neuroleptics produce lower percentages of D_2 receptor occupancy and are less likely to cause depolarization inactivation suggest that other mechanisms of action may also be operative.

Besides EPS, the side-effects of the conventional antipsychotics vary widely across classes and, for the phenothiazines, within classes (see Table 16). Among the phenothiazines, the lower potency aliphatic (chlorpromazine) and piperidine (thioridazine) compounds have the greatest anticholinergic, antihistaminic and anti-α_1 adrenergic activities and the greatest cardiotoxicity. Conversely, fluphenazine and haloperidol are the most potent and selective D_2 blockers; they also have the greatest risk of EPS, and a lower risk of cardiotoxicity or orthostasis.

Suggested reading

Casey DE. Effects of clozapine therapy in schizophrenia individuals at risk for tardive dyskinesia. *J Clin Psychiatry* 1998; **59** (Suppl. 3): 31–7.

Glazer WM. Extrapyramidal side effects, tardive dsykinesia, and the concept of atypicality. *J Clin Psychiatry* 2000; **61**(Suppl. 3): 16–21.

Ho B-C, Miller D, Nopoulos P, Andreasen NC. A comparative effectiveness study of risperidone and olanzapine in the treatment of schizophrenia. *J Clin Psychiatry* 1999; **60**: 658–63.

Honigfeld G, Arellano F, Sethi J et al. Reducing clozapine-related morbidity and mortality: 5 years of experience with the Clozaril National Registry. *J Clin Psychiatry* 1998; **59** (Suppl. 3): 3–7.

Kane J, Honigfeld G, Singer J, Meltzer HY for the Clozaril Collaborative Study Group. Clozapine for treatment-resistant schizophrenia: a double-blind comparison with chlorpromazine. *Arch Gen Psychiatry* 1988; **45**: 789–96.

Kinon BJ, Lieberman JA. Mechanisms of action of atypical antipsychotic drugs: a critical analysis. *Psychopharmacology* 1996; **124**: 2–34.

Marder SR. Antipsychotic medications. In: Schatzberg AF, Nemeroff CB, eds, *Textbook of Psychopharmacology*, 2nd edn, 309–21. The American Psychiatric Association: Washington, DC, 1998.

Marder SR, Davis JM, Chouinard G. The effects of risperidone on the five dimensions of schizophrenia derived by factor analysis: combined results of the North American Trials. *J Clin Psychiatry* 1997; **58**: 538–46

Owens MJ, Risch SC. Atypical antipsychotics. In: Schatzberg AF, Nemeroff CB, eds, *Textbook of Psychopharmacology*, 2nd edn, 323–48. The American Psychiatric Association: Washington, DC, 1998.

Segal J, Berk M, Brook S. Risperidone compared with both lithium and haloperidol in mania: a double-blind randomized controlled trial. *Clin Neuropharmacol* 1998; **21**: 176–80.

Stahl SM. *Psychopharmacology of Antipsychotics*. Martin Dunitz: London, 1999.

Suppes T, Webb A, Paul B *et al.* Clinical outcome in a randomized 1-year trial of clozapine versus treatment as usual for patients with treatment-resistant illness and a history of mania. *Am J Psych* 1999; **156**: 1164–9.

Tohen M, Sanger TM, McElroy SL *et al* for The Olanzapine HGEH Study Group. Olanzapine versus placebo in the treatment of acute mania. *Am J Psychiatry* 1999; **156**: 702–9.

9. Mood stabilizer practical pharmacology

Practical information

What is a mood stabilizer?

The term 'mood stabilizer' has been widely accepted and appears frequently in the psychiatric literature despite the absence of a consensus definition. Although conceptually appealing, the 'mood stabilizer' classification is difficult to define. If the designation were reserved for therapies demonstrating efficacy in double-blind trials for all four of the primary therapeutic objectives only lithium would be included in this category. Such a definition would be too restrictive and impractical. Therapies demonstrated to be effective for one or more of the primary therapeutic objectives may offer valuable mood stabilization to bipolar patients so long as it can be administered without the risk of exacerbating the illness.

For practical purposes, a 'mood stabilizer' could be defined as a treatment that decreases the vulnerability to subsequent episodes of mania or depression and does not exacerbate the current acute episode when administered during the acute, continuation or maintenance phase of treatment. This definition includes in the mood-stabilizer category treatments, which, by virtue of their protection against (manic or depressive) recurrence, result in a decreased rate of cycling whether or not they possess acute antimanic or antidepressant properties.

For any patient, a first-line mood stabilizer would be one that had a desirable safety profile and reasonable efficacy. In practice, this means there is no individual contraindication (known hyper-sensitivity) and the potential for intolerable effects (e.g. seizure, coma, death) is very low and the tolerability of the expectable adverse effects is very high. In the US the FDA has granted approval to lithium, divalproex and olanzapine for the treatment of mania. In Europe, lithium and carbamazepine have regulatory approval.

Lithium salts

Although many medications are believed to have prophylactic mood-stabilizing effects, only lithium salts have been proven to reduce the risk of recurrent episodes of mania and depression by multiple studies using double-blind, placebo-controlled discontinuation designs.

Lithium prophylaxis generally follows acute-phase treatment with lithium carbonate, lithium citrate (i.e. the elixir form) or a controlled-release preparation (i.e. Lithobid® or Eskalith CR450®). Most studies have employed doses that deliver blood levels in the middle or lower half of the therapeutic range (i.e. 0.6–1.0 mmol/l), leading to the convention of 'maintenance doses' of lithium salts. This may result in a reduction in the daily dose of lithium when compared with the acute phase of treatment, which should be accomplished before beginning the maintenance phase of treatment.

The dose and blood level of maintenance-phase lithium therapy is critical for several reasons. On the one hand, many side-effects are dependent on blood concentrations and maintenance-phase therapy at higher blood levels is associated with greater attrition, non-adherence and more complaints of side-effects. On the other hand, very low blood levels, even within the lower quarter of the therapeutic range, have been associated with a greater risk of manic or depressive relapse. Thus determining the optimal dose of maintenance lithium therapies is a collaborative process that evolves over time. Nevertheless, a relapse at a lower blood level certainly provides *prima facie* evidence that a higher dose course of treatment will be necessary in the future.

On occasion, lithium salts may be initiated for prophylaxis during the maintenance phase. For example, another mood stabilizer may have been used in the acute phase but tolerability has become problematic during longer-term treatment. In such cases, lithium should be started at lower doses (e.g. 300 mg, b.i.d.) and titrated against side-effects to achieve blood levels of 0.6–0.8 mmol/l.

Later emerging side-effects of lithium therapy include acne, weight gain, and subtle memory or concentration difficulties. Polyuria, excessive thirst and edema can be problematic and may foreshadow more worrisome changes in renal function. Weight gain may similarly reflect emerging hypothyroidism. Other side-effects, such as sedation, diarrhea or tremor, which may seem trivial immediately following an acute mania, can become more annoying during longer-term therapy.

Many side-effects can be managed by a combination of dosage reduction, shifting dosing to bedtime only or switching the formulation to one of the sustained-release products. Although the patent-protected sustained-release formulations are more expensive than generic lithium carbonate, the very low overall costs of these simple metallic salts is an important advantage when compared with newer alternatives.

Recommended laboratory monitoring during longitudinal lithium therapy is summarized in Table 17. Frequent (monthly) blood level monitoring is usually not cost-effective outside research settings, although it might be considered in response to adherence problems.

Divalproex
In the US divalproex is now more commonly used as acute-phase therapy than lithium salts and, as a result, it is used increasingly as a maintenance treatment. Clinical experience suggests

that divalproex is preferred for the prophylaxis of rapid cycling, lithium-resistant and mixed presentations of bipolar disorder, although definitive controlled studies have not yet confirmed these impressions. Conversely, there is no reason to assume that divalproex is less suitable for prophylactic therapy (when compared with lithium salts) after more classic episodes of mania. It is also likely that valproic acid has similar efficacy, although the enteric-coated divalproex formulation has significant advantages in tolerability.

There is no established blood level range for divalproex associated with better prophylactic outcomes. Generally, maintenance-phase therapy follows the doses used during the acute and continuation phases and results in blood levels ranging from 40–120 µg/dl. The longer-term side-effects of divalproex maintenance therapy include weight gain, hair loss and sedation. When possible, dose is consolidated at bedtime, although nausea and other gastrointestinal side-effects may preclude a complete consolidation despite use of the enteric-coated formulation.

Recommended laboratory monitoring is summarized in Table 18. There is some concern about the possible development of polycystic ovaries during long-term treatment. This concern, which arose from studies of patients with epilepsy, has not yet been confirmed in prospective, longitudinal studies of patients with bipolar disorder.

Divalproex maintenance therapy may be initiated during a sustained recovery if a patient has developed intolerable side-effects or renal changes during lithium therapy. Generally, therapy is initiated at lower doses and titrated slowly (e.g. 250 mg/day) to minimize side-effects until a stable blood level of at least 40 µg/dl has been achieved.

Carbamazepine

Carbamazepine (Table 19) was the most commonly prescribed alternative to lithium salts prior to the introduction of dival-

Table 17 *Lithium.*

Approved indications	Warnings	Drug interactions	Most common adverse effects	Most worrisome adverse effects	Initiation/ maintenance therapy	Laboratory investigations	Patient education
Bipolar mania	Renal impairment	Diuretics	Gastro-intestinal irritation	**Acute intoxication:**	**Initial dosage:** 300–450 mg bid	**Pre-treatment:** CBC	**Expect (one or more):**
Maintenance therapy for bipolar disorder	Cardiovascular disease	NSAIDS	Sedation	Seizure	then titrate to therapeutic range or highest dose tolerated	Electrolytes	Gastro-intestinal irritation
	Complicated fluid or salt balance	Cabamazepine	Tremor	Coma		Thyroid	Sedation
		Ca²⁺ blockers		Death		Creatinine	Mild tremor
	Acute myocardial infarction	ACE inhibitors	**Other:**			BUN	Thirst
	Myasthenia gravis	Metronidazole	Weight gain	**Intoxication sequelae:**		Urinalysis	Increased WBC
	Pregnancy	Neuroleptics	Edema	Renal		EKG if > 35 or clinically indicated	
			Acne	Cardiac			**Report:**
			Psoriasis	CNS		**When stable:**	Moderate tremor
			Polyuria			Li 1–4 months for 1 year then every 4–6 months	Slurred speech
			Polydipsia	**Other:**			Muscle twitching
				Thyroid inhibition			
				Arrhythmias			
				Renal dysfunction			
				Teratogenicity			

Table 17 *contd.*

Approved indications	Warnings	Most common adverse effects	Drug interactions	Most worrisome adverse effects	Initiation/ maintenance therapy	Laboratory investigations	Patient education
					More gradual titration (to minimize side effects): 300 mg qhs for 2 days 600 mg qhs for 2 days 300 mg qam/ 6400 mg qhs for 2 days then 600 bid	**Every 6–12 months or when clinically indicated:** TFT Creatinine BUN Urinalysis CBC	Change in fluid balance Impaired memory Rash Edema **Discuss:** Lab rationale Weight control Importance of sodium Potential teratogenicity

Table 18 Divalproex (Depakote).

Approved indications	Warnings	Drug interactions	Most common adverse effects	Most worrisome adverse effects	Initiation/ maintenance therapy	Laboratory investigations	Patient education
Bipolar mania	Impairment of liver function	**Increased VPA levels:** Aspirin Felbamate Rifampin	Tremor Dizziness Sedation Nausea/ vomiting Gastro-intestinal pain Headache Elevated LFT Somnolence Asthesia Dyspepsia Rash	Marrow suppression Thrombo-cytopenia Prolongation of coagulation time Pancreatitis	**Initial dose:** 250–500 mg bid	**Pre-treatment:** CBC with diff Platelets LFT	**Expect** (transiently): Sedation Tremor Gastro-intestinal symptoms
Prophylaxis of migraine headaches	Blood dyscrasia				**More gradual titration** (this can mini-mize side-effects):	**Follow-up:** Establish level 50–100 mg/l	**Report:** Easy bruisa-bility
Reduce incidence of complex partial seizures		**Decreased levels:** CBZ Clonazepam (rare) -absence status		**Other:** Hair loss Weight gain Teratogenicity Possible association with polycystic ovari-an syndrome	250 mg qhs for 2 days 500 mg qhs for 2 days 250 mg qam/ 500 mg qhs for 2 days then 500 mg bid	Weekly until stable drug level; CBC and LFTs. **Monthly** for 6 months. **Thereafter** every 6–12 months	Abdominal swelling Rash Jaundice Edema (facial)

Table 18 *contd.*

Approved indications	Warnings	Drug interactions	Most common adverse effects	Most worrisome adverse effects	Initiation/ maintenance therapy	Laboratory investigations	Patient education
		Inhibits: Diazepam Lamotrigine Phenobarbitol Phenytoin Weak inhibition: P_{450} isoenzymes			**Alternative rapid titration:** Day 1: single dose 20 mg/kg Day 2–4: split bid Day 4: serum level Day 5: adjust as required for valproate= 80 μg/ml If no improvement in 2 weeks, increase as necessary for valporate = 100 μg/ml		Discuss: Weight control program Common drug interactions Potential teratogenicity Use of vitamins/ minerals (folate, Se, Zn)

Table 19 Carbamazepine (Tegretol).

Approved indications	Warnings	Drug interactions	Most common adverse effects	Most worrisome adverse effects	Initiation/ maintenance therapy	Laboratory investigations	Patient education
Epilepsy	Impairment of cardiac, renal, or liver function	Induces; P$_{450}$ CYP 3A4	CNS Dizziness Sedation	Aplastic anemia Agranulocytosis	**Initial dosage:** 200 mg bid-tid	**Pre-treatment:** CBC with diff Platelets	**Expect:** Sedation Gastrointestinal symptoms
Trigeminal neuralgia	Prior hematological dyscrasia	**Reduces:** Neuroleptic levels	Unsteady gait Cognitive impairment	Thrombocytopenia	**More gradual titration** (this can minimize side	LFT Urinalysis	Lightheadedness
		Oral contraceptive	Blurred vision/ diplopia	Hepatitis Skin:	effects):	**Useful:**	
	History of bone marrow depression	CBZ Many others	Elevated LFTs Gastrointestinal	Rash (puritic, erthematous) Erythemia multiforme	200 mg qhs for 2 days 400 mg qhs for 2 days	EKG Electrolytes Reticulocyte count	**Report:** Rash Jaundice Incordination
	Sensitivity to tricyclic compounds or MAO inhibitors	**Increased by:** H$_2$ blockers Nefazodone Erythromycin Isoniazid Propoxiphene Valproate	Nausea Anorexia Pain Vomiting	or nodosum Toxic epidermal necrolysis Stevens-Johnson syndrome	200 mg qam/ 400 mg qhs for 2 days then 400 bid	**Follow-up:** Every 7–14 days: CBC, drug level, LFTs for 2–3 months and stable dose	Irregular heartbeat Facial edema

118

Table 19 contd.

Approved indications	Warnings	Drug interactions	Most common adverse effects	Most worrisome adverse effects	Initiation/ maintenance therapy	Laboratory investigations	Patient education
		Ca²⁺ channel blockers Lithium CYP 3A4 inhibitors (e.g. nefazodone) inhibit Tegretol metabolism CYP 3A4 inducers, increase tegretol metabolism		**Other:** Hyponatremia Altered thyroid function Edema Arrhythmia or AV block Alopecia SLE Potential teratogenicity	Titrate to clinical response, not level	**Routine follow-up** (monthly for 4 months): drug level, CBC LFTs, electrolytes Thereafter q6–12 months: CBC, drug level, LFTs, electrolytes, TFT	**Discuss:** Importance of weight control program Common drug interactions Potential teratogenicity Use of vitamins/minerals (folate, Se, Zn)

proex. Like divalproex, carbamazepine has been most commonly prescribed for patients who have not responded to or failed to tolerate lithium salts.

Clinical experience suggests that the therapeutic activity of carbamazepine is greatest at doses that result in blood levels of 4.0–1.2 µg/dl; corresponding doses often range from 400–2000 mg/day. When possible, a single bedtime dose is preferred, with persistent sedation, lightheadedness or transient neurologic signs of toxicity (e.g. diplopia or ataxia) occasionally preventing dose consolidation.

Initiation of carbamazepine during maintenance-phase treatment typically begins with a low dose (e.g. 200 mg/day) and slow titration, minimizing side-effects, to achieve a medium-range blood level (e.g. 60–80 µg/dl).

Other mood stabilizers
Gabapentin (Neurontin®) (Table 20), lamotrigine (Lamictal®) (Table 21), olanzapine (Zyprexa®), risperidone (Risperdal®) and topiramate (Topamax®) (Table 22) are gaining acceptance as mood stabilizers but have not yet been studied as longer-term prophylactic therapies for bipolar disorder. The controlled data supporting their use is limited to mostly acute studies and in some cases the data are weak or even negative. Therefore trials with the more established mood stabilizers are warranted before agents with unproven efficacy are offered.

Although some encouraging open experience has been reported for gabapentin, two double-blind studies failed to demonstrate gabapentin's superiority over placebo as a treatment for mania or bipolar depression. Double-blind studies and placebo-controlled trials have demonstrated the efficacy of lamotrigine monotherapy as a treatment of bipolar depression (50 mg and 200 mg/day) and rapid cycling (100–200 mg/day). Lamotrigine was not more effective than placebo in doses tested for treatment of acute mania. There was, however, no evidence of treatment emergent mood elevation or cycle promoting action in any of the lamotrigine trials.

Olanzapine and risperidone have been studied in double-blind trials. Olanzapine (10–15 mg/day) has been shown to be more effective than placebo, and risperidone (2–6 mg/day) added to lithium or divalproex has been shown to be more effective than monotherapy with lithium or divalproex. Based on the data from controlled trials, these agents appear to be robustly effective for acute mania and would be considered mood stabilizers by virtue of the absence of any evidence of exacerbating mania, precipitation of depression or cycle promoting activity.

Topiramate 256 mg and 512 mg/day was studied as a treatment for acute manic and mixed episodes in a double-blind placebo-controlled trial. The results for topiramate 512 mg/day on some outcome measures (Clinical Global Impression) was significantly better than placebo but did not reach statistical significance on the Young Mania Rating Scale.

Omega-3 fatty acid was studied in a 4-month trial in which fish oil (*n* = 16) or olive oil (*n* = 14) was added to the ongoing treatment regime of bipolar subjects who entered the trial in any phase of the illness. Although a survival analysis revealed a statistical advantage for Omega-3 (longer time remaining in treatment), it is difficult to interpret results from this small trial in which the sample was heterogeneous when randomized at baseline.

Finally, recommended laboratory monitoring for tiagabine is shown in Table 23 and a summary of the pharmacological profiles for the mood stabilizers mentioned in this chapter is given in Table 24.

For the mood stabilizer menu of reasonable choices, see Figure 13 in Chapter 5.

Table 20 *Gabapentin (Neurontin).*

Approved indications	Warnings	Drug interactions	Most common adverse effects	Most worrisome adverse effects	Initiation/ maintenance therapy	Laboratory investigations	Patient education
Adjunctive treatment for partial seizures in adults	Impairment of renal function	Antacids	Somnolence Ataxia Fatigue Nystagmus CNS effects: Dizziness Sedation Unsteady gait Inco-ordination Cognitive impairment Blurred vision/ dipolpia	Worsening mania **Other:** Hair loss Weight gain Teratogenicity (category C)	**Initial dose:** 300–600 mg aq for 3–5 days then increase daily dose 300–600 mg each week **Usual maintenance dose:** 900–3600 mg More gradual titration may be necessary for some patients.	None required **If recent pretreatment:** CBC with diff Platelets LFT Urinalysis **Useful:** EKG Electrolytes	**Expect:** Sedation Gastrointestinal symptoms Lightheadedness **Report:** Rash Inco-ordination

Table 20 contd.

Approved indications	Warnings	Drug interactions	Most common adverse effects	Most worrisome adverse effects	Initiation/ maintenance therapy	Laboratory investigations	Patient education
			Elevated LFTs Gastro- intestinal effects Nausea Anorexia Pain				**Discuss:** Importance of weight control program Common drug interactions Potential teratogenicity Use of vita- mins/minerals (folate, Se, Zn)

Table 21 *Lamotrigine (Lamictal).*

Approved indications	Warnings	Drug interactions	Most common adverse effects	Most worrisome adverse effects	Initiation/ maintenance therapy	Laboratory investigations	Patient education
Epilepsy	Impairment of liver function Renal impairment	**Increase lamotrigine levels:** VPA **Decrease lamotrigine levels:** Phenytoin Phenobarbital Primidone Carbamazepine Phenytoin Folate inhibitors	Sedation Insomnia Dizziness Ataxia Nausea/ vomiting	Stevens-Johnson syndrome **Other important effects:** Rash Blurred vision Diplopia Esophagitis Teratogenicity (category c)	**Initial dosage:** 50 mg qd for 2 weeks 50 mg bid for 2 weeks Then increase daily dose 100 mg each week to usual maintenance dose 150–250 mg bid	None required Potentially useful if concurrent with drugs that alter metabolism: Serum levels LFT CBC	**Expect (transiently):** Insomnia Sedation Nausea Dizziness **Report:** Rash **Discuss:** Common drug interactions Potential tratogenicity

Table 21 contd.

Approved indications	Warnings	Drug interactions	Most common adverse effects	Most worrisome adverse effects	Initiation/ maintenance therapy	Laboratory investigations	Patient education
					If concurrent valproate: 25 mg qd for 2 weeks 25 mg qd for 2 weeks Do not exceed 150– mg/day		

Table 22 *Topiramate (Topamax).*

Approved indications	Warnings	Drug interactions	Most common adverse effects	Most worrisome adverse effects	Initiation/ maintenance therapy	Laboratory investigations	Patient education
Epilepsy (Adjunctive therapy for adults with partial seizures)		**Decrease topiramate:** Phenytoin CBZ VPA Oral contraceptive pill Acetazolamide Dichlorphenamide	**CNS effects:** Somnolence Dizziness Anxiety Ataxia Speech disorder Psychomotor slowing Confusion **Gastrointestinal effects:** Weight loss Anorexia	Renal stones	**Initial dose:** Inpatients: 50 mg Then increase by 50 mg each day to therapeutic effect or highest tolerated dose **Outpatients:** 50 mg qd × 7 days then increase daily dose 50 mg each week	**Pre-treatment:** None required **Potentially useful:** Serum levels LFT CBC **Maintenance:** None required **Useful:** Urinalysis Electrolytes Creatinine	**Expect:** Sedation Gastrointestinal symptoms Lightheadedness **Report:** Rash Jaundice Inco-ordination Irregular heartbeat Facial edema

126

Table 22 contd.

Approved indications	Warnings	Drug interactions	Most common adverse effects	Most worrisome adverse effects	Initiation/ maintenance therapy	Laboratory investigations	Patient education
					Usual dose: Acute mania 200–800– mg maintenance dose: 100–600 mg More gradual titration is necessary for some patients.	**Pretreatment:** None required **Potentially useful:** Serum levels LFT CBC **Maintenance:** None required **Useful:** Urinalysis Electrolytes Creatinine	**Discuss:** Common drug interactions Potential teratogenicity Use of vitamins/ minerals (folate, Se, Zn)

Table 23 *Tiagabine (Gabitril).*

Approved indications	Warnings	Drug interactions	Most common adverse effects	Most worrisome adverse effects	Initiation/ maintenance therapy	Laboratory investigations	Patient education
Epilepsy (Adjunctive therapy for partial seizures)	Impairment of liver function Renal impairment	**Increased tiagabine clearance:** Phenobarbital Phenytoin Carbamazepine	Dizziness Sedation Asthenia Tremor Ataxia Nausea Difficulty concentrating	Abdominal pain Confusion Esophagitis Headache Anxiety Teratogenicity (category C)	**Initial dose:** 4 mg qd for 5–7 days then titrate daily dose 4 mg each week to clinical effect or highest dose tolerated **Usual dose:** Acute mania 4–16 mg **Maintenance dose:** 4–12 mg qhs	None required Potentially useful if concurrent treatment with drugs that alter metabolism: Serum levels LFT CBC	**Expect (transiently):** Insomnia/ sedation Nausea Dizziness **Report:** Easy bruisability Rash Jaundice Edema (facial) **Discuss:** Common drug interactions Potential teratogenicity Use of vitamins/minerals

Table 24 *Mood stabilizers – pharmacological profile.*

Drug	Activity				Metabolism					Common forms
	Gaba	Ion channel blockade	Excitatory amino acid	Other	Major pathways	Inhibits	Induces	T$\frac{1}{2}$ (hours)	% Protein bound	
Lithium	↑GABAb	None		PKC Phospho-inositol	Renal excretion	None	None	18–30	NA	Li$_2$CO$_3$ 150,300 mg 300 mg SR 440 mg CR Li citrate 5m^3 = 8 mEQ
Carbamazepine	↑GABAb	Na			Hepatic 3A4	None	3A4	Initial 25–65 Sustained 12–17	75	100, 200, 400 mg
Valproate	↑GABAb	Na	↓	PKC	Hepatic: Glucoronidation Beta oxidation	P$_{450}$ isozymes Epoxide hydrase Glucuronosyl-transferases	None	6–16	40–95	Tablets 125, 250, 500 mg

Table 24 contd.

Drug	Gaba	Activity			Metabolism			T$^1/_2$ (hours)	% Protein bound	Common forms
		Ion Channel blockade	Excitatory amino acid	Other	Major pathways	Inhibits	Induces			
Lamotrigine		Na Ca	NMDA		Hepatic: Glucoronidation Renal excretion	Dihydrofolate reductase	Self	25–30	55	25, 100, 150, 200 mg
Topiramate		Na Ca	AMPA	Carbonic anhydrase	Hepatic: Hydroxylation Glucoronidation Renal excretion			21	15	25, 100, 200 mg
Gabapentin	↑				Hepatic: Glucoronidation Renal excretion			5–7	<3	100, 300, 400 mg
Verapamil		Ca						5–12	90	40, 80, 120 mg
Amlodipine		Ca						30–50	93	2.5, 5.0, 10.0 mg

Appendix A: Example of a daily mood chart

Daily charting

44 y/o Male
cc=Depression

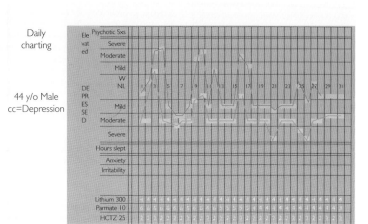

Appendix B: Clinical monitoring form: treatment and symptoms

Name: _____ ID# _____ Others: _____ Physician: _____ CPT code: _____ Visit Type: _____ Date ___ / ___ / ___

Over the past 10 days, how many days have you been/had ...

	% days	Severity (0–4)		DSM Criteria Satisfied	
			No	Probable	Definite

DSM Criteria

	% days	Severity			
...depressed most of day:	— %	—	Depressed most of the day nearly every day for ≥2 wks		
...less interest in **most** activities or found you **couldn't enjoy even pleasurable** activities through **most of the day**:			Decreased interest or diminished pleasure in most activities most of the day nearly every day for ≥2 wks		
...any period of abnormal mood elevation	— %	—	Mood Elevation (high, euphoric, expansive) to a significant degree over a 4–7 day period		
...any period of abnormal irritability	— %	—	Irritability to a significant degree over a 4–7 day period		
...any abnormal anxiety	— %	—			

Rate Associated Symptoms for PAST WEEK

Much more **+2**   **0** = usual/none   **−2** Much less

MDE requires ≥5 (including depressed mood and/or interest)

Depression	Sleep	Interest	Guilt/SE	Energy	Conc/Distr	Appetite	PMR/PMA	SI
—	—	—	— or —	—	— or —	—	— or —	—
	EBT _____ DFA _ MCA _ EMA	Self Esteem	Need for sleep	Talking	FOI/Racing thoughts	Distractible	Goal directed activity/PMA	High Risk Behavior

Sleeps ___ – ___ hours

							LNWL ___ Passive ___ Active	
		DGOOB	Naps	Anhedonia				SI

Elevation
Mania/hypomania requires ≥3 unless only irritable, then ≥4 moderate sxs are required (do not count elevation or irritability) toward dx of hypomania or mania

yes no **New major stressor, if yes** _____

yes no **Significant Medical Illness, if yes** _____

Additional **Psych tx:** OP ER Hosp	Additional **Gen Med tx:** OP ER Hosp

___ c/d caffeine   ___ ppd nicotine

yes no **Substance abuse** ___ d-use/wk   **Onset of menses** ___ / ___ / ___   early   later   **NA**

yes no **Alcohol abuse** ___ d/wk

___ Panic   ___ Binge/Purge   ~ weight ___

___ HA   ___ Migraine HA

contd

Current Treatments

	Dose Mg 24 total	Mg Missed Past 7 days			Dose Mg 4 total	Mg Missed Past 7 days
Mood Stabilizers						
Anxiolytics/Hypnotics						
Antidepressants						
Antipsychotics					PRN	X
					PRN	X

Psychosocial Interventions _____ /mo   ECT _____ /mo   Other _____ /mo

Yes   No   Significant Noncompliance, if yes _____

Comments:

Adverse Effects

Severity 0–4

Tremor	
Dry Mouth	
Sedation	
Constipation	
Diarrhea	
Headache	
Poor Memory	
Sexual Dysfunction	
Increased Appetite	
Other	
EPS	

Selected Mental Status   Severity 0–4

PI _____   IOR _____   OC _____

Hallucinations _____   Delusions _____

Last Labs   **Date** / /

Li = _____   VPA = _____   TSH = _____

Creat = _____

Current Clinical Status (check on)

___ **Depression**	___ **Continued Sxs**
___ **Hypomania**	___ **Recovering**
___ **Mania**	___ **Recovered**
___ **Mixed***	___ **Roughening**

If new episode, estimate onset date: / /

Other Dx: _____

CGI _____   GAF _____   GAF _____
(1–7)   week (0–90)   month (0–90)

Path _____   _____   Phase: A   C   M   T
Path _____   _____   Phase: A   C   M   T

Plan:

RTC _____

133

Index

Note: BPD = bipolar disorder